KILLING CANCER

ONE MAN'S JOURNEY DOWN THE CANCER TRAIL...

L.J. MARTIN

WOLFPACK PUBLISHING
— EST 2013 —

Killing Cancer
One man's journey down the cancer trail...

L. J. Martin

Wolfpack Publishing
6032 Wheat Penny Avenue
Las Vegas, NV 89122

Paperback Edition
Copyright © 2018, 2010 L.J. Martin

Paperback ISBN: 978-1-88533-915-7
eBook ISBN: 978-1-885339-17-1

CONTENTS

KILLING CANCER

Please feel free to pass this book along to any and all who are fighting cancer or who have a loved one fighting this hated disease!

DEDICATION

This journal is dedicated first to my beautiful, patient, concerned wife, Kat, who prodded and cajoled and encouraged all through these ordeals; then to my docs, in both Missoula and Houston; then to all those over the years who've fought the good fight against this rotten disease and sought alternative solutions to whipping it; and last, but certainly not least, to my good friend Mel McGowan, whose fight goes on, and whom I know will win, for good attitude and mental toughness are a good part of the answer. And particularly to Mark Scholz M.D., America's No. 1 cancer killer!

DISCLAIMER

The author is not a physician or a health professional of any kind, he's merely a survivor.

His first cancer was one which takes over 30,000 lives a year in the U.S., prostate cancer, the man's cancer as breast cancer is generally, but not always, a woman's disease, and as uterine and ovarian cancer is exclusive to woman.

The second cancer was squamous throat cancer, with a tumor located in the lymph gland on the left side of his neck as well as a primary tumor on the back of his tongue. A national survey says that only 16% of men between 65 and 70 years of age diagnosed with throat cancer will survive. The author looks at statistics with a skeptical eye.

There's no way to be certain that any of the

herbal or homeopathic treatments he tried had any efficacy on either of the cancers he had, and he utilized every medical professional he could to effect a cure, however, he was cured. The author is not proscribing or even suggesting that these herbal, diet, and homeopathic remedies are in any way to be a replacement for expert medical treatment, and is only offering a frank and candid look at what he did to overcome and cure his cancer, and continue his lifestyle for whatever that may, or may not, be worth.

He is, however, enjoying a healthy, active life today.

KILLING CANCER

INTRODUCTION

by Mark Scholz M.D.
Medical Director, Prostate Oncology Specialists,
Inc., Marina del Rey, CA

Executive Director, Prostate Cancer Research
Institute, Los Angeles, CA
Prostateoncology.com
Author/Editor
The Key to Prostate Cancer
&
Co-Author
Invasion of the Prostate Snatchers: No More
Unnecessary
Biopsies, Radical Treatment or Loss of Sexual
Potency

"GOD HELPS THOSE WHO HELP THEMSELVES"

Getting a life-threatening diagnosis like cancer naturally leads to thoughts about life, death and God. I have often heard Christians criticize the statement above as, "Not being from the Bible." Well, so what? What's wrong with self-reliance?

Maybe the problem is that we humans fall too easily into "either / or" thinking. We struggle to keep two abstract thoughts alive in our feeble brains simultaneously.

The two thoughts I am referring to (as related to finding a cancer cure) are:

1. Work your tail off to find the best doctors and best treatments.
2. Pray like mad.

Christians, being spiritual, are expected to seek answers in the invisible realm first. They fear overzealously pursuing point #1 works to the detriment of point #2.

As a cancer expert taking care of patients for over 30 years, I have indeed noticed an unhealthy tendency. Patients tend to put all their eggs in one basket by over-relying on one doctor, one faith, one type of treatment, or one type of diet.

Cancer, being a vicious foe, should stimulate us to adopt a more mature approach. To use a military analogy, why put all your trust in a single smart bomb? Do we think we are smart enough to pick the magic bullet with 100% certainty? The sensible approach is CARPET BOMB the enemy!

Patients who are suddenly thrown headlong into a cancer diagnosis can't realize the type of challenge they are facing. The medical system is stacked against their getting the latest and most up-to-date treatment. Medical systems in the US (and throughout the world) strongly lean toward using older, less effective treatments rather than newer ones. Why would that be?

1. In this modern era of galloping technological progress, it is *the norm* for doctors to be unfamiliar with the latest developments. No one can keep up.
2. Insurance companies push doctors to use

older treatments because they are far less expensive.

3. Busy doctors are more comfortable with familiar, older therapies because they are less likely to trigger malpractice suits.

4. Doctors don't like use cutting-edge treatments for fear their peers will label them as quacks. The Catch 22 is that treatments are only deemed totally safe after becoming widely accepted. Realistically, the timeline for broad acceptance of a new therapy requires 10 to 15 years!

Both Larry and I are passionately concerned about patients who passively accede to a dumbed-down authoritative medical system whose major focus is protecting itself. Patients who just want to get along and avoid making waves will be cheated out of receiving the best available treatment.

In this highly entertaining book, Larry vividly relates his pathway to victory over two life and death battles with cancer. This book is a wonderful, real-life illustration of how powerful it can be to adopt an aggressive, "I can do this" type of spirit. Larry's true story of perseverance, courage, and out-of-the-box thinking is the perfect prescription for patients who want to KILL THEIR CANCER.

PREFACE

KILLING CANCER: ONE MAN'S JOURNEY DOWN THE CANCER TRAIL

October 2018

I'm now over eight years cancer free—if any of us really know that our body is cancer free. My friend Mark Scholz, and in my opinion, the world's expert on prostate cancer, who I still see twice a year, has been kind enough to write an introduction to this work. I'm indebted. The fact is had I known of Dr. Scholz when I originally discovered I had prostate cancer, my approach to treatment might have been different. Medical treatments evolve and improve, thank God, He and many great research scientists and physicians. Mark Scholz is an oncologist and my favorite kind of doc...an open-minded one. I'll never forget him and those in his practice saying, basically, if it ain't broke don't fix it. Otherwise if you're doing something that is working, even if only God can understand why, don't be in a hurry to try something else. But pay careful attention.

That said, you can't look backward. Or go back in time. We don't, as of yet, have a time machine. If this little tome doesn't do anything else, I hope it convinces you to be assertive about your health. You're the only one living in your body and your awareness may give you many, many extra years.

June 2009

It started, this time, with a knot not much larger than half a child's marble, just beneath the jaw on the left side of my neck. An infected lymph node...I hoped... however already being a cancer survivor I was not one to wait to see what transpired. Even though an infected lymph node is often associated with a fever blister, and I was just getting over my first blister in several years, I wanted to know for sure.

A call to a local head and neck medical center resulted in the typical: "The doctor can see you in five weeks." I laughed, if a bit sardonically, not only thinking, but saying, "I could be dead in five weeks!" Didn't help. Was I being a hypochondriac? I hoped so, but I was more than happy to be thought one for the peace of mind. But more so, I was convinced I had to be proven one by a thoughtful, professional, diagnostician.

If this journal helps you in any way, I hope it convinces you to be proactive about your health. It's not some smiling receptionist at the doctor's office who'll have to go through the long, lonely, and oft times rocky road of your cancer. It's you, and in the final analysis, only you, who'll have to deal with it. If you take no for an answer, then you can only blame yourself if you don't stop the monster in its tracks. And even if you get in to see the doc, be skeptical. I can't begin to tell you how many stories I have of misdiagnosis. Medicine is a science, but it's not a perfect science. It's oft times an art as well. You want your doctor's best educated guess, but you want it backed up with hard science if he/she, or you, have any doubt.

Doctors' won't be my primary audience for this journal as docs hate patients to self-diagnose and particularly to insist on tests docs think unnecessary. The internet has to be the bane of their existence, for too much information is spread so easily…of course much of it is erroneous.

And we all seem to be ruled by what the insurance companies or Medicare will pay for. Just because we, or even our doctor, believes a test is in order, the insurance company or Medicare may disagree, and worse, the doc may be influenced against even prescribing a test because he thinks they won't pay. We have for some time—and I fear the problem will grow to horrid proportions in the future —been subject to bureaucratic medicine, i.e., bean counters dictating your care.

In my case…no, I'll fill you in on my current case when I get to that part of the journal.

I'm starting this journal while it's my wife's turn driving—we travel a lot, usually for much more enjoyable reasons, usually researching one of our novels, and each drives for a hundred miles while the other reads or writes, as I'm doing now. We're on our way to the University of Texas M. D. Anderson Cancer Center in Houston, Texas, a two thousand mile drive from home in Western Montana. It's been almost a two month odyssey from feeling a knot in the neck to pointing the car toward Houston.

Why two months? Why so far away to be treated? I'll answer those, as well as other questions, as this journal moves forward. The basic reason is an odyssey to find the best health care in the world. But, who knows, maybe it'll be my wife who has to finish this report as this is a disease whereby even the best may not be good enough.

I THINK THOSE TWO MONTHS AFOREMENTIONED are critical if you want at be a cancer survivor rather than a cancer victim, so I'm going to belabor the past eight weeks, and the path leading through them, and through my prior bout with cancer and its aftereffects. The rest of this journal, after this historical intermission, will be written while I'm going through a rather intensive, both mentally and physically, treatment for squamous cancer, evaluated as a stage four by a couple of the docs I've seen, but stage three by most of them...and I choose to believe the latter, of course, as the treatment goes for a cure of stage three, and only "buys time" for stage four.

One of the lessons of this journal is not to wish for a thing too much, or for the exclusion of a thing too much, or either might just happen. In this case, I hated, in fact obsessed about, tongue cancer...and guess, in this my second bout with cancer, where my primary tumor turned out to be? A dear friend of mine died just one year before from a head and neck squamous, one month from the time it was discovered. That was almost my undoing then, and gravely affects me now.

We're all touched by cancer, the monster with many faces. I recently read that 41% of us will develop cancer at some time in our lives and many of those will die from the disease. So even though you may be healthy, and may think I'm only preaching to the choir here, I'm not. Cancer touches all of us; if not you, then someone near and dear to you. One might begin to believe that we're doing something wrong in this wonderful country of ours?

My first bout with one of the serpents slithering from Medusa's ugly head came years ago, at the age of 52. I'm 77 as of this revision. Had I been truly cancer aware, I would have been overly concerned about having a problem holding my water. I put the slight incontinence problem off to age...until while madly searching for a bathroom in an unfamiliar town where my wife and I were doing a booksigning. I hurriedly left the store with its unusable, out-of-order, restroom to find one that worked, and finally when I couldn't hold it and watered my levis while still in the car, I desperately pulled into an alley. I concluded the job among the trash cans at the risk of being hauled in for indecent exposure. And I felt indecent, and worse. I had to wait until my pants dried before I could show myself in public again. Humiliating? You bet. An ominous sign? You bet.

But it wasn't until a couple of weeks later, when I developed a persistent ear infection and a lesion on my arm, neither of which seemed to be healing, that I decided to go to the doc.

Now I know when things don't heal it's likely because your bodies fighting something far more important in another location.

Dr. Alverez had a clinic not far from our condo in the central California city of Bakersfield where I was born and where my wife, Kat, migrated from a much smaller San Joaquin valley town. He'd been suggested by a good friend, because she knew his receptionist and she would get me in.

The clinic was full of Mexican field workers and their families and not being fluent in Spanish I felt a little out of place, however, it was clean and efficient appearing. And this wasn't a big deal, an ear infection and a sore that wouldn't heal and those symptoms hardly call for a visit to a major medical facility —I later concluded that my body was busy fighting bigger battles elsewhere, using its assets elsewhere, and ignored these less important interlopers. And I even later concluded that a big fancy office doesn't necessarily mean the best care. I kept in touch with Dr. Alverez for many years, and although I haven't spoken with him for quite a while, he still remains warm in my heart. I hope he's happily retired with his favorite fishing pole or golf club in hand.

Pay attention to the warning signs your body gives you. With cancer you don't want to wait and see. I did however wait my turn to see Dr. Alverez. The doc, whom I immediately liked, was attentive and treated my symptoms, each of which quickly went away in the next week. He gave me a complete physical, including running his index finger up my backside to palpate my prostate. This, of course, is SOP for a man's physical exam and happened another half dozen times in the next couple of months. Having a twisted sense of humor, it was hard not to respond "yes, darling," when asked to turn around and assume the position. He found no symptom with the finger exam, nor did any other examiner thereafter. But more importantly he recognized the threat and suggested a PSA blood test; a relatively new test at the time, common now. I liked him because he was attentive, and because he took on all comers, regardless of social status or of how deep were their pockets. He was a healer, in the fine old sense of the word.

It was a short few days when his office called and wanted to see me. He reported that I had a PSA of 89...not .089 or .89, but 89. I, of course, didn't know what that meant, but I was damn sure going to find out.

I did know that he referred me to a urological surgeon for a biopsy of my prostate.

Experience is a wonderful thing...it enables you to recognize a mistake when you make it again.
The definition of insanity is doing the same thing over and over again expecting a different result.

2

BEING A WRITER BY PROFESSION, I'D OFTEN USED
the over-worn analogy of "as much fun as a
root canal."

A prostate biopsy is as much fun as a mouthful
of root canals. But mostly because of where it's
located; it's intrusive and embarrassing, but the
slight pain is over quickly, and as with most
medical procedures the fear of it is far worse than
the actuality. That said, having a couple of large
male hands working in your mouth is one thing,
having them in your rectum is altogether another.
Actually, the procedure's done with a small tube
apparatus that's inserted into your rectum, then,
when a trigger is pulled, shoots a needle through
the wall of your colon into the target, your prostate,

gleaning a few cells as a sample to be evaluated by a pathologist. Usually they take at least four shots, one to each quadrant of the prostate. Again, the procedure's demeaning and humiliating, and a little worrisome.

The thought of perforating your colon, probably the least sanitary portion of your digestive tract, from the inside out in order to investigate other parts of your body is disconcerting to say the least.

One thing you learn quickly is to overcome all thoughts of demeaning and humiliating when you're trying to save your life. It was three days before I learned that that was exactly what I was doing.

One of the longest, most agonizing, times in your life is awaiting the outcome of a biopsy. But the outcome arrived. Prostate cancer. Not only prostate cancer, but a virulent form. Prostate cancers are rated on a scale called a Gleason. I presume that's named after the lady or gentleman who developed the process. Gleason ratings are 1 through 10. Mine was a 7. Not the worst of prostate cancers, but considered well above the norm and very aggressive as prostate cancers go. That, along with the mere fact it was a cancer, was even more disconcerting. Frightening is a much more accurate word. And, oh yeah, my father died of prostate cancer.

Once you overcome the shock of the result, then it's time to reconnoiter and circle the wagons.

I knew something about prostate cancer, at least from a layman's standpoint, as my father had died just three years prior to my diagnosis. What I knew of it was all bad. He died very hard, and even though I didn't know him from the time I was seven years old until I was in my twenties, still, one is deeply touched by the loss of a parent. He liked John Barleycorn better than he liked us for those early years, and for a few thereafter. My father and I got to be good friends in the years following, after he became good friends with AA, but it never quite leaves your mind that he wasn't there when you were growing up... however, I wish I'd treated him better, spent more time with him when he was ill. If actually having cancer teaches you one thing, it's empathy.

But back to the problem at hand. Later, post prostate biop, I would have a cat scan, an MRI, and an ultrasound, which turned out to be another rectum invader. The ultrasound is (or was) preformed with a long tube, the diameter of a man's index finger, attached to a cord which is in turn attached to a monitor and recording machine. To my way of thinking, it's a little less than manly to have a long cylinder inserted in your backside...in fact there's a term for men who participate in that as recreation. I found it way less than appealing and it will never follow my thoughts about, "what are we doing for fun today?" And of course, it's demeaning and humiliating...again.

All of the above, however, are part of most prostate cancer regimens, so you bite the bullet and grab your ankles, figuratively if not literally.

And of course, there were needles. Needles didn't particularly bother me then, nor do they now. And it's a good thing. I've probably had at least a hundred pokes, mostly for the determination of PSA.

MRI's, on the other hand....

It wasn't too many years later that I developed an acute case of claustrophobia. No matter how much I worked on my mind, on getting my mind right...you know, repeating "this is going to save your life,"...no matter how much I thought my mind was right...I'd still try and tear up a very expensive machine trying to evacuate that tunnel shortly after they rolled me into that much too small a space. Yes, you have some room if you are not overly large, but it felt like being mummified to me, closed in on me like the slamming of a crypt's iron door. You might as well embalm me first.

As it turned out, later in life, when and if an

MRI was necessary, I simply advised, "knock me out." I had two subsequent MRI's under that blissful condition.

To demonstrate how claustrophobic I was, a radiologist and good friend of mine gave me an injection which he said, "knocks anybody out." When I remained wide-eyed, he gave me another. When I still steadfastly remained wide-eyed, he exclaimed, "I've never had to administer more than two." And gave me another. This time, I didn't even remember him pulling the needle out. The next thing I knew it was forty-five minutes later and I was trying to pull my boots on, but I had not tried to destroy his very valuable MRI machine, and the procedure was completed successfully, and, thank God, the result was successful as well.

But I digress. So, I had prostate cancer.

What to do?

Never be afraid to try something new...remember a single, dedicated man built the ark.
A team of experts built the Titanic.

3

My newly acquired urological surgeon said, of course, "We must operate. A radical prostatectomy." It's common for surgeons to believe that "A chance to cut is a chance to cure." And it often is the only chance. But I asked, what does that mean? A radical prostatectomy? And he said, to my great chagrin, after dancing around the potential results of the surgery for some time, and insisting that it was the only way to save my life, that it meant no erections and no ejaculations. I was five years married (after three years living together) to a very desirable woman who at forty-five—she looked thirty-five or younger—was seven years my junior, and we were still, very sexually active. We liked and were attracted to each other. Sex was a large part of our attraction. Both of us had been married before. I loved her and couldn't conceive of living without her, or even with her without that part of our relationship. There had to be another option.

I've never been one to accept a single opinion, seldom in business, but particularly when it's my life, or even my sex life, that's at stake. So I thanked the nice surgeon and said "I'll get back to you."

When I was first advised by Dr. Alverez of my PSA, which I learned referred to Prostate Specific Antigen, I turned to a relatively new resource, the internet. By the time my biopsy was reported, I had a one foot deep stack of information on prostate cancer. I certainly was no expert, but I was rapidly becoming an informed layman (of course you're easily also mis-informed on the web). Among many other things, I learned that there was a so-called 'radical operation' and a so-called 'nerve sparing operation' to remove the prostate and its parasite. There were also lots of other alternatives: cryogenics, implanted radioactive seeds, etc., etc., etc.

THE RADICAL PROSTATECTOMY removed all chance of a normal erection and both radical and nerve sparing operations removed the ejaculation as the prostate produced the semen that was the liquid carrier of sperm, produced by the testicles. I had, by the way, had a vasectomy many years before, already being the father of four sons from my first marriage— there was some speculation at the time that a vasectomy contributed to the onset of prostate cancer, but that notion seems to be dismissed. The nerve sparing operation could leave you with the blood supply necessary for a normal erection, thus making sex possible. That's the good news. The bad is it also left you with a much greater chance for the return of the disease—return is probably the wrong word as it's actually a greater chance of missing some cancerous cells, thus not solving the problem. So it wasn't returning, it could just be somewhat missed.

EVEN WITH THE ability for an erection, what was sex for a man without an ejaculation?

DID I HAVE A MILLION QUESTIONS? That's probably a conservative estimate. What was the risk of a nerve sparing prostatectomy? If the risk was too great, would it be worth trading a short life and possibly painful lingering death for enjoying a sexual relationship for that short time? Was it even fair to expect my wife to continue to have sex with someone whose sexual organs were, or had been, infected with cancer?

As it turned out these and the other 999,997 questions were moot.

One of my favorite stories:

At his retirement party, a man was approached by his son, who said, "Great that you're retired dad. Are you gonna go fishing?"

"No, son, I'm thinking about going to law school."

When he quit laughing, the boy said, "Pop, law school takes three years. In three years you'll be 68."

THE MAN PLACED a hand on the boy's shoulder and looked concerned, then offered. "Gee, son, you're right. I hadn't thought of that."

THE BOY LOOKED SATISFIED, then the man added, "by the way, sonny, in three years how old will I be if I don't go to law school?"

4

When I returned to the urological surgeon for the "follow up" he said flat out that no surgeon would agree to a nerve sparing operation when my PSA was so high. It has long been my mantra, "never say never."

For most of my early life, the first twenty five years of my working life, I was a salesman. Even though I was a licensed real estate broker, building contractor, and appraiser, and was active in those disciplines, I still considered myself a salesman, and was proud of the fact. I had long lived by the proposition that nothing happened until someone sells something. Sales drove the engine that was and is this great free enterprise system of ours. And salesmen, at least the great ones, don't take no for an answer. And I also knew that even experts don't always arrive at the same conclusion. Medicine, as I said, is a science, but also an art. Art, many times, in fact all times, is subjective.

Of course I wanted to live, but I wanted to live a full life with my beautiful, sexual, wife, who, by the way, was rapidly becoming one of the nation's leading writers of woman's romantic suspense and historical romance. Romance was never far from her mind. And, after long consideration and many conversations with her—even with her repeating time and time again that all that was important was that I stay alive—I was willing and eager to take the risk...if I could find a surgeon who would perform the nerve sparing operation.

When I walked out of that first surgeon's office, I made up my mind that one opinion was certainly not enough. I certainly was not the first cancer victim to want a second opinion. I was going to go to the best, at least in the west, and I'd listen and learn, but I would make up my mind quickly as time is the enemy of one with a cancer diagnosis. All the while you're trying to make up your mind what tact to take, your cancer is consuming both oxygen (so I'd been told) and glucose at ten times the rate of normal cells, and growing without consideration of other structures in your body.

I was not, however, going to jump into the common solution (the first thing a doc tells you to do) without having the facts.

The first fact is that doctors, like all of us, don't like to lose. They much prefer to err on the side of caution. And to those who aren't willing to gamble with life, even if it's someone else's life and/or quality of life, caution is the only route to take. Not a bad approach, and it undoubtedly saves a lot of lives, but how much quality of life?

I've always been, admittedly, hedonistic. I've always looked at life as a great trip, and you might as well take the high road. Work hard, play hard, make some money from hard honest work, and have some fun spending it…and maybe save a little for your old age so you won't be a burden on others. When I first proposed marriage to my wife, Kat, I did so with the proviso, "We may not make a lot of money, but we'll have a lot of fun." And that self-serving, gratuitous attitude, unfortunately, followed through with my dietary habits. Why self-serving? I ate what pleased me, not what was serving my health. Why gratuitous? There was no payment, no health benefits from my diet, or at least very little.

The fact was my hedonism showed in many ways. I ate, and drank, what I wanted, and didn't eat what was merely good for me. We enjoyed lots and lots of red meat and had wine with every supper, I loved fried foods, and we usually met with friends for a few drinks every Friday.

We didn't have much money when I was first diagnosed with cancer, but we did have health insurance, which expanded our options. I didn't have to take potluck when it came to being treated. I had recently made a little money in the real estate business, prior to plunging into the writing life, and, thank God, my wife was a much better money manager than I. It was thanks to her much more conservative approach to life that we had health insurance. We'd both ventured into the writing business, which is about like saying we were depending upon hitting the lottery. We'd had some publishing success, but it was yet to translate into real money; still hand to mouth. I was not unaware that I owed her for her good sense in insisting on health insurance.

Suddenly, it came to me that I was not indestructible. Life was suddenly not quite the lark I'd taken it for. The lark had flown.

So, the hunt for a surgeon who'd perform a

"nerve sparing prostatectomy" was on. And hunt we did. USC, Stanford, Scripts, University of San Francisco, and eventually UCLA. At the same time we were visiting these university hospitals, I was on the internet looking for new innovative solutions, hoping against hope that a less invasive solution, less sexually destructive solution, was available. And there were lots of new things being done, but none of them with a track record of success that would satisfy us. I was also on the phone talking with major medical facilities all over the nation. Nothing hit my hot button.

On calling UCLA, not far from our home in Bakersfield, I was assigned a surgeon to speak with. Dr. Erlich had just expanded his practice from pediatrics to adults. He had small hands, which he'd have to have to operate on tiny children (or at least so I thought), and working inside the body is tight work, and he was very intelligent and quick witted. He understood my need to retain some sexual function, and agreed to do the nerve sparing operation with the proviso: "We'll see what we can do when we get inside." Which was all I'd ask anyone to do, and I hadn't asked any of the surgeons for more than that. He was the only one who'd even broached the possibility of sparing some nerves and blood supply. All the other surgeons (I think it was seven by this time) had said unequivocally they'd only do a radical prostatectomy.

The ultrasound I'd already received showed the cancer protruding outside the prostate, a protrusion described as the size of the first joint of the thumb. Not a good sign for it not having metastasized to other organs.

Your friends love you anyway.

5

THE SURGERY WAS SCHEDULED FOR TWO MONTHS, November, at the UCLA Medical Center, a teaching hospital as were the other university hospitals. Losing my prostate was to be my happy Thanksgiving...and saving my life was surely that.

So now the quest was to beat the cancer into submission as best I could, and that, to me, meant the best diet and exercise regimen I could accomplish.

I had been a cook all my life, having started cooking at the ripe old age of eight. My brother, Rex, and I were raised by my mother after my dad found John Barleycorn a better companion than the three of us. Mom had to work. My brother, four and a half years my senior, decided that we would cook so she didn't have to when she returned after a hard day's labor. I can't tell you how impressed I was when he (with my help as dumb labor stirring his mix) made a cake. It was our first attempt at pleasing her with even a piece of a meal, and she was so pleased (being a great mom she at least acted as if she was) that we decided we'd cook dinners, and often did. My brother is still an excellent cook, and I ended up cooking my way, as a cafeteria fry cook for fifteen hundred hungry students, through college (at least until I had to leave my junior year). I've had a couple of restaurants in my day and cooking has been both a vocation and an avocation.

Cooking anything was not a particular problem for me. However, changing my diet from the BBQ to the juicer was a major transition. During my study of the disease, I decided that diet was a major factor in the cause of cancer, and still believe so. I decided that the fastest way to pack my body with the vitamins, minerals, enzymes, and other nutrients it needed was to juice—using a kitchen appliance to remove the juice from fruits and vegetables—and juice I did. I bought a Jay The Juiceman juicer and consumed 70 ounces of fresh juice everyday. The basis of what I did was carrots and apples (at Jay's recipe pamphlet's suggestion), which gave a decent flavor base to whatever else I added...and I added damn near everything that graced the green grocer's shelves. Beet's, turnips, rutabagas, peppers, ginger, etc., etc. I used so-called organic items if I could find them, but that was before the serious craze for non-toxic foods. If it was edible and had some liquid, I shoved it in the juicer. I also became much more faithful at going to the gym. I stayed very light on the red meat and stuck with fish and chicken. In a month I felt as strong as a bull. I'd lost those ten extra pounds and was down to fighting weight. If only I could meet the cancer in a back alley and get it on... unfortunately cancer is a sneaky underhanded bastard and doesn't fight fair and seldom out in the open.

One of the side effects of a prostatectomy was incontinence. I gave myself a quick course on how your body controls the flow of urine, and decided exercise would help with that. There's a muscle which in a man is a figure eight, encircling the anus and the urethra. Where it circles the urethra it's called the urethral sphincter. During urination, the bladder neck opens, the sphincter relaxes and the bladder muscle contracts. Incontinence occurs if closure of the bladder neck is inadequate (stress incontinence) or the bladder muscle is overactive and contracts involuntarily (urge incontinence). In a woman the muscle's a double figure eight, with three structures being encircled, the third being the vagina.

Like any muscle, exercise would improve it. Contracting that muscle where it circles the urethra is how one voluntarily cuts off the flow of urine. It's simple to identify as it's the muscle that contributes to tightening up the anus. So, I did three sets of a hundred puckers, or extreme tightening, every day. Try it, it's not as simple as it sounds, and it certainly improves the ability to cut off the flow of urine. I had very little problem with incontinence after my operation.

By the way, no physician ever suggested such an exercise.

What I didn't know at the time was that, with the juicing of vegetables, I was keeping my body in an alkaline PH state. I thought I was merely giving my body everything it needed, when in fact I was depriving it of something it didn't need...acid. I'll go into this much more later, after my journey though the long and rocky road of prostate cancer. And my later fall from grace.

So when the day came to report to UCLA, I was as physically fit as I could be in that short time.

The good surgeon spent over four hours inside

my lower belly (twice as long as he said he'd be), which upset my waiting wife and friends, but turned out to be a good thing. When I awoke, and was wheeled to my room, my beautiful wife awaited and reassured me that the doc had reported that my "margin's were clear" and that everything went well. They biop the lymph glands in your upper inner-thigh to determine them to be free of metastasized disease. And mine were. I presumed that meant that the cancer hadn't spread, and that seemingly turned out to be the case.

But how about the "nerve sparing" aspect. I had to await the appearance of the surgeon to get that question answered.

When he did appear, he informed us that the extra time the surgery took was the intricate work to try and save all the nerves and blood vessels he could. His evaluation at the time was that he'd saved 70% of the nerves and blood supply that both gave feeling to sex and drove the process of erection. There was a good chance I could have normal sexual relations, sans ejaculation. I, being a man, had already spent a lot of time wondering about how normal sex could be without ejaculation.

The other good news was I was healthy, and set a record, at that time, of getting out of the hospital following a prostatectomy. I credit that to juicing and exercise, and of course to the hospital: the nurses and doctors great care. To give you a hint about post-op hospital release, the criteria seems to be a bowel movement and your ability to stay off pain medication. After the second day being hooked up to a pain medicine delivery machine I got smart. The machine had a button you pushed if you felt you needed pain medicine, and it beeped upon delivery via the IV tube in your arm. I learned later it beeped none the less with a push and only delivered the pain medicine on a given schedule, no matter how many times you pushed. The psychosomatic result of pushing the button and hearing the beep was positive, even though you might be being tricked.

I, no matter how good the food or how pretty the nurses, asked when I got to go home. The nurse informed me of the bowel thing and the pain thing, and I immediately said, "get rid of this pain med machine," and they did. I had to wait another day for nature to take its course. Then I started yelling "let me out of here." And they did on the morning of the fifth day; now almost everyone is out in three (maybe even less now), so I've lost bragging rights.

Of course, I was still carrying a catheter and a bag. Because of the fact they bisect your urethra, a very tough tube that carries your urine from your bladder to the outlet; it has to have a chance to heal before the catheter can be removed. In ten days or so I returned to have the catheter removed. Because the surgeon wanted the catheter to remain absolutely stable, he'd wired it into the bladder. The wire actually was doubled and extended through the bladder wall and through the stomach wall to the surface, where it was secured with a coat-sized button. I looked a little like a rag doll with a button on my belly. After a couple of days, no matter how much powder and lotion you use, you're ready to get rid of a catheter. The end of a man's penis is not where he wants to develop a rash that you couldn't touch with a powder puff without eliciting a wince. However, let me tell you, it's a bit of a thrill when the doc nips the wires free from the button, and with one energetic pull jerks those double wires back through your stomach muscles, the bladder, out through the urethra, and through a very surprised penis—happy to be rid of the intrusion of another tube, but surprised. I don't get too wide eyed as a rule, but you could see the whites of my eyes for several minutes after that experience. I hadn't asked about the process in advance, and sometimes it's better not to do so. This was one of those times.

As a preventive measure, the doc wanted me to undergo 35 days of radiation. Being an early riser I made arrangements in Bakersfield to get my treatments at seven AM every weekday until I'd completed the process. I worked every day and had no adverse effects, other than a little weariness, from the process.

I was cancer free, or so I hoped and prayed, and in a couple more weeks was able to test my radically revised equipment.

Nobody cares if you can't dance well...
Just get up and dance.

6

I WAS NOT PARTICULARLY THRILLED TO DISCOVER that 70% is not quite enough to have satisfactory sexual relations. Before the operation what I had I would have referred to as a "whiskey hard-on." Inferring that having drunk too much a man couldn't perform.

Again, not to be discouraged, I began to look for solutions to that problem. And again, there were a number offered. We settled on the easiest and less intrusive of the many "pumps" that were available, including internal ones, to achieve a respectable erection. In this case it was an external tube with a suction pump, hand or battery operated—available with a prescription for about four hundred bucks or in any sex shop for about sixty nine dollars and ninety five cents. The good news is it worked (works) well—I'm happy to say I've worn out two of them (more now, I'm happy to say). The bad news is it takes a good deal of the spontaneity out of the event. Still, not a bad trade when you consider no sex, or an operation to install an internal pump that still needs to be activated (an internal bulb pumped by pressing on the groin), as the alternatives.

Of course there was always the alternative of a permanent prosthetic that kept you in a state of erection at all times. I thought that might prove a fashion challenge but didn't need to spend a lot of time worrying about it as my wife nipped that idea in the bud, so to speak. It seemed the occasional mechanically induced erection was enough for her. It reminds me of Mae West saying "does he like me or is that a banana in his pocket?" I presume she was not high on every woman thinking I was interested.

It helps, and in fact is imperative, to have a good woman by your side, and I had the best. We never lost our sense of humor, and it was a good thing as I'd promised her "we may not make a lot of money, but we'll have a lot of fun." And we continued (continue) to do so.

I believe that besides diet, and faith, laughing is cancer's worst enemy.

The fact was I could have sex without the pump, but it was much more satisfying to me, and to my ego —and I'm sure to her though she'd never say so—for me to have an erection so hard the cat couldn't scratch it. Okay, that's a blatant exaggeration. Still, it was functional.

Subsequent to that time they've developed an operation to bypass the normal blood supply to the penis by bringing it from another source. To be truthful, I don't feel the need to spend the money or put up with the aggravation, and am happy with the mechanical apparatus. I was surprised, however, that the loss of a good portion of the nerves didn't seem to affect my enjoyment, the physical sensation, of the event.

The best news of all is, like female orgasm, male orgasm without ejaculation is just as satisfying as with...and a lot less messy. I was astounded to find that my orgasms lasted longer and in fact were more satisfying. You couldn't wipe the silly grin off my face.

Sex, at least with one you love, actually is an emotional thing as well as a physical one. It's amazing what a man learns as he grows older. It's said that a woman needs flowers, candy, and a candlelight supper, and all man needs is a place...but it seems there's actually a lot more to it, to both emotionally and physically satisfying sex, than that.

Post prostatectomy your PSA should remain at zero. If all the prostate was successfully resected, removed, then there should be no tissue to produce Prostate Specific Antigen. Again, I'm no physician, but that's as I understand it. So if you have a positive PSA reading, then you either have some prostate tissue left, or you have some cancer left, which also is capable of producing PSA.

My PSA began to rise a couple of years after my operation. I let it go as high as .10. Normally, docs begin to get concerned when it goes over .05, which is considered the high end of normal for a man with a prostate. Not good news. As additional surgery was out of the question—we'd been told that post radiation surgery was not possible—I set out to find the best urologists in the business, and settled on a couple of docs at Marina Del Rey in Southern California. They immediately put me on Lupron and Casodex. One of which required a daily pill, the other a monthly injection. The good news was my PSA retreated to zero, the bad was, after a year or so on the medication, my body began to change. These medicines are, as best I understand it, to remove a man's testosterone, the primary hormone that makes

33

a man a man...and that feeds prostate cancer. P.S. I'm now on Casodex alone and doing very well—no physical changes, PSA remaining near .01.

I began losing my body hair, and I'd always been a hairy devil, and, to my great shock, my boobs were beginning to grow. Like most men I enjoy a great set of boobs...but my own? I think not. I got off the medicines, and stayed off for eight months...until my PSA began to rise again. Back on the prescription drugs. Off again in eight months. The PSA began to rise again. Back on the prescription drugs. This time I vowed to stay on them for a year. I did so, even though I didn't like what they were doing to my body.

The medicines didn't seem to affect my sex drive, thank God. So I stayed on them the last time for a full year, then quit. My PSA remained at zero for almost a year, then again began to creep up.

I can't begin to tell you how many cancer victims I know who have outlived their doctors who said, "Sorry, but you'll be dead in six months.

7

DURING THIS WHOLE PROCESS, I CONTINUED TO scan the web, looking for alternative ways to drive the PSA down, thus, hopefully, any risk of the return of the cancer—although secretly, I thought it was hiding out somewhere in the old body and had been ever since it was first discovered. The body is, needless to say, an intricate mechanism, and there are lots of places for a few cells to hide.

My PSA had risen to about a .07, wherein most docs would be looking at the prostate for a serious infection, or for prostate cancer, when I stumbled on a paper written by a University of San Francisco doc, one considered to be among the top urological guys in the State of California (by this time we were living in Montana). He described an herbal formula that was prepared by a California company. He'd done a study on forty guys with non-responsive prostate cancer (did not respond to normal testosterone deprivation treatment), some of them with much, much higher PSA's than mine had been before my operation, and twenty seven of the forty had gone to zero PSA. To me, particularly at that time, it was revolutionary for a physician to even look at an herbal (botanical) solution to any kind of disease. The product was PC Spes, non-prescription of course, and I immediately ordered some. The maximum dose was suggested by the company to be eight tablets a day, and I immediately began that regimen. In four months, my PSA was zero.

It was said to me those many years ago that U.S. doctors received, in medical school, about a half hour of study on alternative cures i.e. herbal medicines. That always came as a surprise to me when so many of the prescription drugs they commonly use are herbal based; as much as twenty five percent of prescription drugs sold in the U.S. are plant based. Some eighty thousand plants are used around the world as treatments. Herbal treatments are the primary health care in China. Who knows what the efficacy of those are? However, it was the primary method of care for many, many thousands of years before the U.S. was the U.S. We do know that digitalis, aspirin, quinine and other drugs spring from plants. The opium poppy is the basis of morphine in all its medical (and heinous) formulations. The list goes on and on.

In Germany, to the contrary, one third of all graduating doctors have studied herbal medicine and a medical therapeutic guide to herbal medicines has long been published there.

PC Spes was formulated from saw palmetto, licorice, reshi mushroom (known as the long-life mushroom in China), Baikal skullcap, rabdosia, Dyers woad, chrysanthemum, and Panax ginsing. Who knows what curative value those ingredients have, or what the combinations thereof have? All I know is that my PSA went to zero.

To the credit of my docs in Marina Del Rey, who had prescribed the Lupron and Casodex, when I reported the efficacy of PC Spes to them they responded, "If it's working, keep it up." Not all physicians are so open minded and pragmatic.

I can only speak from experience. I stayed on that formulation for about four years, until the State of California shut down the production of PC Spes. I did try and get off the pills twice during that time, and twice my PSA began to rise. Back on, PSA zero. To me, the proof of the puddin' was in the eatin'.

The state and other cancer scientists claim to have discovered prescription medications in the formulation of PC Spes. And I don't doubt that they did find some chemical composition that either was, or closely resembled, prescription drugs. Those drugs were not listed on the label, and even though PC Spes made no claims to curing cancer, even herbal supplements must reveal, on the label, their contents.

I have no doubt that the above law is a good one. A company should have to reveal the contents of concoctions they sell. I also am not a chemist, but I do know enough about chemistry to know that many times when you combine substances or chemical compositions other chemicals are formed. Could this be what the state discovered in PC Spes? Something formed by the unplanned, natural, combination of the ingredients? Could this contribute to the efficacy of PC Spes? Something contributed to its banning, no matter how many were helped.

I also have no doubt that the multi-billion dollar drug industry is very jealous of any supplement that seems effective against the same illnesses and diseases upon which they spend hundreds of millions of dollars to perfect medicines to treat, and many millions more to get those concoctions approved by the Food and Drug Administration. I also know without any further investigation that companies who spend that kind of money, and an equal amount on advertising, are very, very powerful. Could they drive a small company out of business should they desire? I don't think there's any question.

This journal is neither being written to try and solve the health care problem in this country nor to provide me with a soapbox to rail against drug companies and what I believe their advertising does to negatively affect all of us. So that's the end of my flailing at windmills.

I will tell you that after PC Spes was no longer available, I did a simple thing. My number three son lived in Seattle, a city with a large thriving Chinese population. I made a list from the PC Spes label, emailed him, and he went to the Chinese herbalist and bought me a quantity of those plants, barks, mushrooms, herbs, etc. When I received them in Montana (a large box), my PSA had begun to rise again. As I recall, it was .04. In addition to the coffee grinder I already owned, I bought another just for the purpose of grinding my new batch of twigs, blooms, and fungi. Within a day I had my witch doctor's concoction. I made tea and drank four to six cups a day. It was not unpleasant, in fact I came to enjoy it as much as I would any green tea. In three months my PSA was again zero.

I extended my middle finger to the health officials of the State of California and the executives of the drug companies. I stayed on the tea for almost three years without any rise in my PSA, until another product, an over the counter supplement, Prostisol, hit the market. I have no question that it was a copy of PC Spes formula with the exception it had a couple of additional ingredients. I immediately picked it up off the internet, placed my faith in it, and my PSA remained at zero. Twice I tried to wean myself from Prostisol, and twice my PSA started to rise. Again, the proof of the puddin' was in the eatin'.

Many docs will tell you that herbal supplements merely "mask" the symptoms of the disease you're trying to defeat. After three years of using prescription drugs to great detriment to my appearance and manhood and finally changing to herbal supplements, I don't even bother to argue with them. The fact is, herbal supplements worked far better for me than did the debilitating and disfiguring prescription drugs.

Recently, one of the great proponents of Prostisol, Dr. Kurt Donsbach (a chiropractor and herbalist) has been arrested for practicing medicine without a license, or so it was reported on the web. Could the drug companies be at work again? I don't yet know the outcome of that arrest, but do know (from press reports) that he was contacted by an FBI agent purporting to be a cancer victim, and arrested when he proclaimed that Prostisol had helped thousands of cancer victims. We're not allowed to bait bears in Montana, and I wonder if law enforcement should be allowed to bait in that manner? I did go to the trouble of contacting his website to offer to testify on his behalf as to the efficacy of Prostisol in my individual case. I don't know the outcome of that arrest, but do know that his website is still active (as of the date of this original writing 2009) and he's still selling herbal supplements.

Will I go back to the tea when and if my PSA begins to rise and I can't get Prostisol?

You bet. (I'm currently on Casodex and doing well)

Am I suggesting that you don't follow doctor's orders? No, certainly I'm not. In fact I'm following doctor's orders, doctors whom I've chosen very carefully, but I'm always looking....

Here I am again facing the monster cancer. And

you know I'm embarrassed about it as I think had I followed my own methodology and not "fallen off the wagon," had not fallen prey to that old hedonism, I would not be here in Houston getting ready to face the death rays (hopefully death to the cancer and not the host), but more about that now....

When the going gets tough...
the tough get going.

8

As soon as I felt the knot in my neck, as I mentioned earlier, I called a head and neck clinic and was advised it would be five or six weeks before the doctor could see me. Sometimes anger is a good thing, and this made me angry. So how to resolve the problem? I had a couple of friends who were physicians, the closest being a back-asswards relative in that his niece had been married to my son. Although she and he didn't remain married, my wife and I considered the doc and his wife among our closest friends. He was a well respected semi-retired orthopedic surgeon.

I called him, knowing a referral would get me in much faster. He was vacationing in Hawaii, but took the call. Upon my explaining my symptoms, he phoned in the referral to the head and neck clinic and I was scheduled to see them in two days time. If you have a problem, and don't know have a doc as a personal friend, I'd suggest you hot foot it to a "doc in the box," one of the clinics in a shopping center, and get a referral from them if possible. The head and neck clinic was curious as to why I was referred by an orthopedic surgeon.

I gave them a smile and a "he didn't like the knot on my neck."

I was not to see the head and neck surgeon but would be seen by his physician's assistant. My appointment was for 4:00 PM. The young man who saw me, Josh, was efficient and impressive. In short order he asked when I could go to St. Patrick's Hospital for a "fine needle biopsy" and a "cat scan."

I asked if "now" would be soon enough.

Before I go on to explain why I ended up in Houston being treated, I want to compliment my adopted home town of Missoula, Montana, and assure my friends and the medical community there that I respect them for the quality of care and the empathy and attention they pay to everyone in need of help. I couldn't have been better treated by the docs and by every employee of docs and hospitals I came across, with one exception. Had I been treated there until the resolution of this disease, I would have gone every step of the way with great confidence. I don't know where else I would have been seen by the cat scan crew and the pathologist the same evening as the need was expressed by a physician's assistant. I'm indebted to all of them.

The cat scan was simple as it only involved from mid throat (base of tongue) to the sinuses. It took a very short time, even though I had to have a I.V. in order to inject dye and I presume in order to quickly administer some kind of anti-reactionary drug should I have a bad reaction to the dye. The whole process was probably less than an hour and a half.

Then it was off to see the pathologist. A so-called "fine needle biopsy" is a bit of a misnomer, at least in my case. My small knot in the neck was by this time the size of a half a walnut. Yes, it was a fine needle, however, If the good doctor stuck me once, he stuck me twenty times. I was not in a lot of discomfort (I tolerate this kind of thing pretty well, having learned to laugh my way through pain, thanks to my older brother's good example), but I thought my poor wife, who'd been at my side all the way, was going to pass out and become the object of the doctor's attention. We were home later that Wednesday night, somewhat worn out.

It was disconcerting that I awoke the next morning with a knot the size of half an egg where the half-walnut had been.

Shrouds don't have pockets and you've never seen a hearse followed by a Brink's truck. Do what you have to do, spend what you have to spend so you can live out your life. Leaving your kids money YOU'VE worked hard for is doing them no favors. There've been more fish caught with a willow pole than all the Orvis rods ever built, and fruit you've picked yourself is always the sweetest.

9

I prayed the increase in "tumor" size was the result of the multiple stabs the tumor had received. And as it turned out, I can only presume the increase was due to a hemotoma—a collection of blood due to injury from multiple stab wounds. But it would take days for that to be proven by the shrinking of the knot back to the size it had been when the biopsy was performed.

We left the next day, with our 5th wheel trailer, for a four day outing on one of Montana's beautiful lakes, north of where we lived. We were taking two of our grandsons, Michael, 14, and Cody, 9, up with us before the weekend to assure a camp spot and my oldest son, Mike, and his lady were to join us on Friday after he got off work. The following day, Friday, my 14 year old grandson, Michael, and I headed for the golf course. I was on the 12th fairway when I received the call from Josh, the physician's assistant, that the result of the biopsy was in and that I had a 2 cm squamous tumor at the base of the tongue that had metastasized into a lymph node on the left side of my neck. The neck tumor was described as 2.5 cm x 2 cm. I finished that hole with a par, better than my usual game, then the wheels fell off and my game went to hell.

I BEGGED off finishing and Michael and I headed back to camp to let Kat, my wife, know that we were in for a battle.

As a QUICK ASIDE AND testimony to the quality of care and empathy shown by the Missoula, Montana medical community, where else would you have received a call immediately after the results of the biop were in? Humanity is still a great part of care in the medical community of Missoula, Montana.

It was devastating news as I'd lost a dear friend to a squamous cancer a year before. He passed one month from the day he was diagnosed. He was a hospital administrator of a very large hospital, and should have had the best care available.

I thought a lot about him on the drive back to the campground, and about his father whom I'd known. We'd been friends since the beginning of high school. His father, upon being given a short time to live, got his things in order, sat in his favorite easy chair, and with all his insurance policies, property deeds, bank accounts, etc., lined up in good order on the kitchen table, along with a letter to his wife, ended his life with a heart shot from a handgun. Not having religious convictions against such an act, I'd always admired him for that, for not putting his family through a long drawn out, expensive, debilitating, depressing, and probably agonizingly slow death. He cheated his disease of that. He thumbed his nose at it, and I think Charley did the right thing and showed a lot of courage and empathy for his loved ones.

I HAD no reason to believe that I had more than a month to live—particularly since the size of the "tumor" had more than doubled in the last few days. Or at least I perceived it had.

When life hands you lemons, make lemonade.

10

I truly thought my time on earth was severely limited. However, I had no intention of dying a long slow death and putting my loved ones, or myself, through that excruciating experience.

I went so far as to call my sons and my brother, and after informing them of the problem, told my brother (who flies his own plane) and those sons close by that my wife might need them in short order as if the disease began to win, I was not going to leave this world a skeletal frame (as I'd watched in the case of both my grandmother and father) in a fetal position or like a sniveling dog—not that either my grandmother or father did so. I loved my family too much to put them through that. I asked my brother to stand by for my call to ask him to fly up, and if he received that call he'd know what it meant without further explanation.

But I also had lots to live for. I enjoyed every aspect of my life. A beautiful house in Montana, another on the keys of a harbor in central California. And the much greater reason of a beautiful wife whom I'd planned to grow old with, as well as four sons and five grandsons and a beautiful blossoming granddaughter. Yes, there'd been stumps in the road, but other than this lump in my neck and on the back of my tongue, I was healthy. Which is a little like saying except for the bullet on a trajectory to take you between the eyes, you're in great shape.

I decided to both get ready to live, and to get ready to die.

I began a draft of a letter (we writers work in drafts) to my wife, I bought stickers to mark things I wanted to give to my sons, personal things that my wife would have to get rid of at some place and time. She'd have little use for my rifles and handguns, my cameras, my computers, and other male things. I had a few collectables and knew the ones she valued, particularly a block of four Pony Express Stamps and a pair of antique pistols. Other collectables of mine she'd have little use for. So, when it came down to the short strokes, I'd mark to whom I wanted things to go.

But at the same time, I attacked the problem by spending hours on the internet studying squamous cancer and what was being done to treat it, and again, changing my diet while cursing myself for letting my diet turn toward those things that only pleased the palate over the last few years. Long gone had been the juicing and the fortifying my body with the great vitamins, minerals, enzymes, and other nutrients gained there from.

I knew from past experience the value of a proper diet, yet I'd been too hedonistic to stay on the straight and narrow path. Meat, eggs, milk, bread, cereal, and sugar made up the majority of my diet. Yes, there was occasionally fruit at breakfast and always a vegetable on a supper plate, a slight nod to good health, but it wasn't always consumed and it took up maybe 25% of one meal of the day. Hardly the seven portions of fruits and vegetables recommended for each day. Not even close.

I immediately bought another juice machine and put it to work, as well as embarked on a herbal regimen I liked based on an old Ojibwa medicine man's herbal mix. Although the general medical population would have disdained the herbal remedies, it was a mixture that had been endorsed by John F. Kennedy's personal physician and he'd often written and spoken about it. That substance is marketed now under many names, and of course none of them make claims to "cure cancer." There are, however, hundreds of testimonial letters about the efficacy of the mix. I bought it as Flow-Essence, compounded by a French company to the exacting standards of that old Canadian First-Nation (Native American to us) medicine man.

During this time I was living on fresh vegetable juice and was losing weight. The docs are concerned when you lose weight and have cancer. I assured them my weight loss was productive. In fact I weighed about 186 when I got the results of the diagnosis. My blood pressure was about 175 over 90. In two weeks on the juice I weighed 172 and my blood pressure was 138 over 70. In this instance, losing weight was obviously healthy. I now keep my weight at 176 or less and weigh daily to make sure I'm not gaining.

My first hours on the web were less than encouraging. A government website said a man between 65 and 70 had a 16% chance of surviving 5 years with a head and neck squamous. It made one want to turn off the computer and go stick one's head under the pillow, or maybe in the oven. But I plowed on. I'm sure those odds are better today, 2018, as they are with most cancers.

"Beginners and outsiders are open to possibilities and don't make assumptions. By extension, they're often better at finding solutions the experts have stopped seeing."
Michael McMilllan
MotivationInAMinute.Com

11

THE NEXT STEP WAS A MEETING WITH THE actual head and neck surgeon. Dr. Haller was well respected in town, and as I understand it, in the west. He'd taught at two universities and "could have gone anywhere" to practice. As an aside, we're fortunate in Montana in that a lot of great docs come there to practice because they love the outdoors and to fish and hunt. He examined me with a method I came to dislike, but one that would become SOP for both surgeons and oncologists. I have a well developed choke reflex, and sticking a finger down to the base of my tongue to palpate the small protrusion there just wasn't something I could tolerate. If fact, the urge to knee the perpetrator in the balls was difficult to overcome even if unproductive.

The next step was to take a look at the tumor. This was accomplished by deadening the nasal passage with a spray and running a small tube up through the passage and down to the back of the throat. I presume the deadening agent was some type of lidocaine as it tasted like...well, I'm not going to say what it tasted like, just rest assured it was distasteful. The tube was a light-transmitting fiber optic cable with the picture observed either with an eye piece on the doc's end, or a flat screen monitor. I was never offered the opportunity to see the monitor and it was probably just as well.

Dr. Haller then made three appointments for me. One with the oncologist or chemotherapist, another with the radiologist (both at St. Patrick's Hospital), and a third to meet him at Community Hospital for a day surgery—a biopsy of the tumor on the base of the tongue. I had actually encouraged that procedure as I didn't want them burning out a cyst thinking it was a cancer. Dr. Haller had already ruled out operating to remove the cancer as he said it would be "far to debilitating." Even if successful, I'd have to learn to swallow and to talk again. And he was encouraging about radiation and chemo, saying, "We'll burn that right out of there."

It was vacation season, and the radiologist was a

stand in for the lady to whom I'd been referred, but the meeting went well and I was impressed with the substitute doctor, also female. She did a fairly complete physical exam, including a finger up the rectum to check, for the hundredth time in my life, my prostate...in this case where my prostate had resided when I had one. Since this was a woman, I decided against my normal "yes, darling," when asked to turn and bend over the table.

With my wife again in the room, the doc explained in some detail and with great patience what radiation would entail. I already knew it meant burns to the exterior of the neck and cheeks and the probability that some weeks into the treatment I very likely wouldn't be able to swallow. Should that happen I would need a feeding tube, either through the nasal passage or via a "peg" in the stomach. After all, they were burning the base of the tongue enough to rid it of a tumor that was now 2 cm plus the margins and would likely be larger by the time treatment actually started.

She did inform me that I couldn't receive radiation to my face without having all dental work, now needed or anticipated in the next few years, completed. It seems the radiation severely inhibits blood flow to the jaw. A rotten tooth that had to be extracted post radiation would leave a hole that would not heal, in fact could cause a bone infection that also would not heal, and could be fatal. The teeth become particularly susceptible to decay as saliva is one of the great deterrents to tooth decay, and another side effect of radiation is the destruction of your salivary glands. Forever after I would have very limited production of saliva, a condition called dry mouth. I would also loose a good portion of my taste, which should return after six months to a year. As the dental work was a factor that could keep me from being treated, we again didn't wait for a referral and resolved to attack that problem in the first available moment.

From there we went to meet with the oncologist, another lady doc. She explained the alternative treatments to us. The worst was a period (up to three months) of weekly chemo prior to beginning radiation, then weekly during radiation. That method would involve a permanent stint near the collar bone, a valve if you will, that stayed in place during the three month treatment. The second alternative would be a weekly visit only during treatment utilizing a vein or I.V. Whichever method I would be given would, most likely, result in my being ill from the treatment. The first, very ill, the second, less so.

My obvious question was, "If this cancer has metastasized to my lungs and liver, does any of this matter?"

The reply of both radiologist and oncologist was "we don't think it has." I was not satisfied with that and insisted upon a lung x-ray and CT scan, which I quickly found was the wrong term. What I wanted was a PET (positron emission tomography) scan, a full body look at what was going on other than in my tongue and on my neck.

The last thing I wanted to do was to put myself through treatment when it was of no use because the cancer was already rampant in my body.

I also posed the question to the oncologist, "Can you kill this cancer with chemo without radiation?" She replied, emphatically, "No."

M. D. Anderson can be reached at:
www.mdanderson.org
713-792-2121
The University of Texas
M. D. Anderson Cancer Center
1515 Holcomb Boulevard
Houston, Texas 77030

12

PET SCANNING IS A HIGHLY SPECIALIZED imaging technique that uses short-lived radioactive substances to produce three-dimensional colored images of those substances functioning within the body. These images are called PET scans and the technique is termed PET scanning. It provides information about the body's chemistry not available through other procedures. CT (computerized tomography) or MRI (magnetic resonance imaging), techniques look at anatomy or body form, whereas PET studies metabolic activity or body function. I had both the PET scan (with the help of valium, closed eyes, and my iPod) and a lung x-ray and both were clean.

My resolve to beat this cancer kept increasing

with each dollop of positive news.

Strangely enough, about this time I received a call from Montana Fish, Wildlife, and Parks, informing me that I'd drawn the super moose tag. To those of you who are non-hunters, this will mean little. One of my primary motivations for moving to Montana was the outdoors; to hunt, fish, and use my cameras. Each of about twenty hunting zones in the state issue, via a drawing, one or more moose tags. The tag I'd drawn was one of one; only one issued in the state via a special drawing. The only tag that allowed you to hunt anywhere in the state for a moose. It was a 1 in 10,000 chance. It was just one of many reasons I had to beat this monster and live on. I'd been putting in for a moose tag for twelve years, and never expected to get this one. It's a one in twenty lifetimes tag. You couldn't get the smile off my face for days. And I'm a guy who's entered hundreds of fund raising drawings and hardly ever won a thing. The good Lord taketh away and the Lord giveth.

The next step was the day-surgery biop of the tongue.

I am not a virgin when it comes to operating rooms. I've had my jaw busted twice (no, not talking when I should have been listening: football and water skiing), both my Achilles tendons severed in two separate instances (playing tennis and playing racket ball), the last digit of a finger torn off (water skiing), and, of course, my prostatectomy. So this small intrusion into my throat only gave me passing anxiety. It did, however, give me a hell of a sore throat, I presumed a precursor of things to come.

Radiation to the head and neck requires absolute dead on targeting. When your tumor rests next to the carotid artery which supplies blood to the brain, and the spinal cord is very close, a millimeter or less is the tolerance. You don't want the machine to be off target or you may not get up off the table, or you make walk away only to suffer an aneurism of the carotid and bleed out before anyone can get to you. Consequently, you must be fixed to the table by a mechanism that keeps you in place...exactly in place. This is accomplished via a form fitting mask beginning at the shoulders and wrapping completely around the head. It's "pegged" down so you cannot move.

Enter claustrophobia again.

I cannot teach anybody anything.
I can only make them think.
--Socrates

13

We attacked the dental problem.

I appealed to the dentist's office where we regularly had our teeth cleaned. Dr. Noah Peter's agreed, under the explained circumstances, that he would see me immediately. He discovered a small cavity, another under a crown, and the fact that a root canal had only been partially completed. He immediately attacked the cavities, pulling the crown and preparing for a replacement, and made arrangements for me to see an endodontist who would complete the root canal. He also launched into a quick study of the effects of radiation as it relates to dental care. Noah was one of those great medical guys who would rather err on the side of caution, and his immediate thought was to have all my molars pulled.

His statement was "three for sure," but all of them if I wanted to be double sure. Remember, pulling all your teeth takes you out of the realm of the dentist, so this certainly wasn't a monetary decision on Noah's part. He wanted what was best for the patient. He also made a cast for a set of trays, rubber receptacles that fit the teeth and allow you to give yourself a fluoride treatment. This would be a nightly exercise for the rest of my life, as the loss of saliva means rapid tooth decay if not treated. (I've now long quit the fluoride and my teeth remain healthy)

Before you repel at that thought, it was, not so long ago, the regimen to pull all the teeth when you were going to have radiation to the mouth area. As I mentioned before, the blood supply to the jaw is radically affected and an infection there can kill the patient because it may not heal. Noah's care was excellent and I would send my grandchildren to him, the best testimony I can give as to how much I thought of him as a dentist. I agreed to consider having all my molars pulled, but to get other opinions. He thought that a good idea.

This is a good time to suggest to you that any medical professional who discourages you from getting another opinion has been a mistake to visit in the first instance. A medical professional should welcome your suggestion about getting second opinions.

On to the endodontist. Dr. Alan Rauckhorst agreed to, under the circumstance, to stay late and see me. Another Missoula medical person who performed above and beyond the call of duty. And again an excellent experience and one that makes me reconsider using "as much fun as a root canal" as an analogy in my writing. With the exception of coming down from the Novocain or whatever pain killer he used, it was pain and irritation free. I inquired as to his opinion about pulling teeth prior to radiation. He performed a complete exam and concurred with Noah that three molars should definitely be pulled.

The criteria here is not teeth that are in need, today, of removal. The criteria is teeth that may be trouble makers in the future. My wisdom teeth were long gone, having been pulled when I was in college. One problem tooth, No. 30, (lower right next to the last molar, No. 31) was not a surprise to me. Several years before a dentist had recommended that he pull that tooth as it had a possible crack and bone loss at its base. I instead elected to visit a specialist in California and have a bone graft. It continued to serve me well for several years. But x-rays showed some cloudy areas again at its base, possible infection, so it had to go. Molars 15 and 17, the last two on the left side, both top and bottom, had gum test depths of 8's. That was considered unacceptable so they were among the doomed.

Not being particularly excited about losing those two molars just because the gum pockets were deep, I elected to visit a periodontist, a specialist in gum disease, Dr. John (Jack) Ramine, who I respected a lot as he'd cared for Kat a number of times. Dr. Ramine, like the others, agreed to see me immediately, and fit me in between patients. He gave me a complete exam and x-rays and concurred that No. 30 was a sure thing and that No. 15 and 17 would be problems in the future, and had to go. He was kind enough to appeal to an oral surgeon, who agreed to have me come in early the next morning.

After arriving at the oral surgeon's at 7:00 AM and receiving a little happy juice and I awoke to find myself missing three teeth.

Your body will tell you that you have a problem, like cancer. Don't ignore that knot where a knot's never been. Don't ignore an infection that won't heal. It may mean your body is using all its resources fighting something else, somewhere else. Be PROACTIVE about your health. After all, you know your own body, or should, better than anyone else.

Above all, don't fear finding out what the problem is. You can't fight until you know the enemy. And the faster you get to the battlefield, the better chance you have of kicking ass.

14

THE GOOD NEWS: AS SOON AS MY MOUTH HEALED
I'd be ready for radiation. The bad: dental work is
not covered by Medicare, even if it's prescribed by
the doctor for a condition that is covered—at least so
I'd been told. I'm still investigating that assumption.
I'd seen four dental experts in as many days. And
still had an appointment to return and get my
new crown.

By this time the knot under my jawbone was
beginning to recede, but of course my mouth was
sore as hell as was my throat from the biopsy. As I
learned, my Dr. Haller had actually taken three
biopsies in my throat, so there were three wounds
there.

My weight had stabilized at 172, which is about

what I should weigh. Now the challenge was to keep it at "normal."

Still, as the knot fell, my sprits rose. It wasn't growing as if it was going to consume my head in a month. In fact, it was going back to the size it was when I began to fight nutritionally with my juicing and witch doctors brew.

I did liberalize my eating, and went back to meat and some wheat products, but kept it at the 25% of the plate to meat and the rest to vegetables.

In my reading, I'd come across a lot of literature on the PH of the body. A PH over about 6.75 is alkaline, and under that it's acidic. There is some widespread belief that an acidic body is cancer's playground. As turns out, most vegetables are alkaline. Red meat is very acidic. Interestingly it is said to take 20 times as much alkaline intake to the body than acidic intake to offset, or neutralize, the acid. Maybe what I'd been doing by juicing with my first bout with cancer was, in fact, increasing the alkalinity of the body?

In order to assist my body in maintaining an alkaline state, I consumed a lot of Essentia ® water, with a very high 9.5 PH. That, and increasing my vegetable intake seemed to do the trick. It was, however, very easy to slip back to an acidic condition with any increase in sugar or meat. High PH water is now available in lots of stores.

Maybe what our mothers and grandmothers have been preaching for generations, "Eat your vegetables," was the best health advice we could have been given?

The sea has historically been alkaline (although I understand that's changing in many parts of the world) and as we all crawled up out of the muck some eons ago, it's said our bodies were alkaline to begin with. And of course, meat was a luxury for many, or most, of past generations. We were hunters, yes, but mostly gatherers, and were nomadic. I've often joked that men are better at directions than women because when we were wandering the plains with our families in tow, the men were shading their eyes and looking at the distant skyline for game, while the women, being far more practical and wanting to make sure there was something for the pot that night, kept their eyes on the ground, gathering plants and tubers.

Women, I think we'll all agree, are still better at details.

No, I haven't given up coffee. I make my coffee with a high 9.5 PH water in order to help offset its acidity.

15

We returned to the radiologist for my mask fitting, which involved me being placed on the table, with a riser under my neck which caused my head to be thrown back, a generous dose of valium helped in this process. A sheet of flat plastic is heated then placed over your head and shoulders and form fitted, to dry. It's designed to hold you exactly in the same place each time it's pegged down to the table. Then, without you getting up, with the mask in place, you're rolled into the machine and a CT is performed. After that, the computer is programmed so each pass of the death ray hits in exactly the right spot.

The mask is made of a plastic that slightly resembles a colander, or a very heavy woven sheet with holes large enough to admit air and some light. It's abnormal for them to cut eye holes and I insisted on those and a mouth hole. I envisioned myself getting ill and upchucking as a result of chemo with nowhere for the material to go. I could reach some of the pegs holding me in place and I imagine I could force myself up to pop the mask free and be able to escape. But I knew the cure, chemo, was going to make me ill. The last thing I wanted to do was aspirate vomit into my lungs, thus causing a problem that might preclude me from being treated for a long period of time. I insisted on a mouth hole.

Being claustrophobic, I knew this mask and "lock down" was going to be a nightmare. I bought a "paint ball" mask, which was the most confining mask I could find, placed myself prone on my wife's treadmill walking-machine, put my head in a waste basket, and practiced staying there for 20 minutes. I gained confidence that I could do this without running screaming from treatment, or tearing up the equipment trying to escape.

I'm sure I'm a physician's nightmare as it seems I'm constantly negotiating with them. However, I'm a fair engineer having gone to school in architecture and having been a builder for a good portion of my work life. Using a piece of paper I demonstrated to them how weak a flat surface was, but how strong it was when you allowed it to curve, as the mask curved. A hole affects the strength very little in a curved surface. The crux of it was I would get my mouth and eye hole as the mask retained its strength, hole or not.

I never got to try that particular mask out under actual treatment.

My brother phoned and suggested I call a mutual friend who had gone through a head and neck squamous treatment at M. D. Anderson.

One of my oldest and dearest friends was an oncological surgeon who specialized in head and neck, however he was retired, and worse, he'd taken a bad fall and was himself recuperating from serious head trauma. He had enough trouble and I didn't want to call him and pour more black paint in his already gray bucket. He had trained at M. D. Anderson and I certainly respected his knowledge and ability, and he'd often said there was no place to compare with the Houston, Texas hospital.

As it happened I had already thought of getting an evaluation there, but it was many, many miles away, and I wanted to be treated where I could go home every night after treatment to lick my wounds in my own surroundings. So I had dismissed the idea.

Kat, too, thought I'd be much better off at home.

I did call the mutual friend in Bakersfield and probably the best and most encouraging thing that happened to me was the fact that, three and a half years post treatment, he answered his cell phone and was in Phoenix watching his daughter play in a volleyball tournament, and sipping a tall cold one. He couldn't have been more encouraging about M. D. Anderson, and his cancer had been worse than mine was thought to be. What better recommendation than sipping a tall cold one, enjoying your family, three and a half years after treatment, and being considered cancer free.

I was given another boost in moral.

Then my dear friend, the surgical oncologist, called, having heard of my problem. His words, I believe, and he's not prone to swearing, were, "Get your ass to Houston!"

Each year U. S. News and World Report magazine does an in depth study of hospitals and their specialties and rates them. M. D. Anderson has consistently placed in the top of cancer treatment hospitals in the nation. This does not mean that there are not other fine cancer treatment centers around the nation, and probably the world. You should seek out the treatment center in which you believe, and in which you and your family have faith.

16

We knew little about M. D. Anderson other than it was renowned for its cancer care and was located in Houston, Texas. A quick "driving directions" search on Google indicated it was a 2,013 mile grind. We had some air miles saved up, so Kat immediately jumped on the internet and began looking for a flight as I jumped on to see what the process was to be seen, evaluated, at the hospital.

It was still first and foremost in my mind that I would be evaluated by M. D. Anderson to get a second opinion and to make sure my docs in Missoula were on the right track.

M. D. Anderson, I quickly discovered, is one of the few medical facilities that has a "self referral" form on their website. No battling for a referral. If you think you need to be seen, you fill out the forms. After my experience at trying to be seen locally, that process brought a smile to my face and a certain sense of faith that the Houston hospital was big, but not nearly as supercilious as many smaller local institutions. It took a couple of days for them to get back to us, and of course we couldn't make travel arrangements until we knew when I could be seen. Shortly we received a package in the mail with date, time, and place to report. I later discovered that my good friend, the oncological surgeon, had called and referred me as well.

I had some limited experience with Houston as my two younger sons lived there with their mother and step-father for some time, and I'd flown in to visit with them. My recollections of the city were not particularly good. I remembered hot, muggy, and bad roads, but I was not going there to vacation so all that mattered little. As it turned out, I came to admire and respect the city and her people.

We got a date to show up, without much explanation as to what would transpire other than, after a phone call: "It will take several days, plan on being here a week. Bring your records."

That was a bit of a shock as I pictured walking in and seeing an expert in head and neck cancer, who would evaluate my records, and after discussing Missoula's protocol with him, getting verification they were on the right track, going home to be treated.

We were scheduled for a Monday, ten days hence.

We immediately began collecting my medical records. I'd had a lung x-ray, CT, and a PET scan and those would be important. I'd also had biops of both the lymph node and the tongue, and a surgical report on the day-surgery for the tongue. As I mentioned before, you should worry about any doctor who doesn't encourage you to get a second opinion, and I'm happy to say none of my Missoula doctors discouraged me in the least. My records were immediately forthcoming.

I did have one problem before leaving, and that was a bone fragment poking through my gum where one of the teeth was extracted. I walked into the oral surgeon's office and was shown to an assistant after a short wait. She informed me that it would "heal over." I informed her that I was about to undergo radiation and if it didn't "heal over" there could be serious complications. She basically shrugged. I left and called Dr. Ramine, the periodontist. He agreed to see me immediately. He got me right in, sat me down and without a Novocain shot, pulled out one piece of loose bone and drilled another "bone spur" down well below the gum line so it would, in fact, heal over. I left with renewed faith in Dr. Ramein and a bad taste in my mouth for the oral surgeon, pun intended.

This disinterest on the part of the oral surgeon's assistant was the only bad experience I had with any Missoula medical personnel. I won't be recommending that surgeon as it's my belief that the buck stops with the boss.

I continued to juice, use my Ojibwa brew, and exercise to try and at least discourage the cancer from growing. It's my belief that exercise is doubly important when you're putting "good stuff" in your body. It opens all those tiny capillaries to that "good stuff" when you get your heart rate up and the blood pumping.

I continued to get ready to live and get ready to die, although my head was on much better as we were doing positive things. How positive? Only the trip to M. D. Anderson would tell. My self-referral had been answered and I'd been assigned a liaison person. Communication is all important when you're in the throes of worry about your condition and about your treatment options. I'd like to say it was easy to communicate with M. D. Anderson but it took some persistence to get answers...but I had an appointment and would be seen. We felt a little like we were charging into a deep dark tunnel, but, hell or high water, we charged on.

Trying for the next few days to live my life normally, I worked in my garden, wrote, messed with some video clips, took care of the yard, went to dinner with friends, and played a little golf. If I told you I didn't occasionally awake in a cold sweat in the middle of the night, I'd be lying, but all in all, I was relaxed considering the circumstance. I also had a few quiet conversations with my maker, hoping he understood that I was a long ways from perfect and I probably needed a lot more time on earth to perfect that state of being. In any case, I wasn't ready for a trip, either up or down. I could only hope the good Lord agreed.

Having had cancer before, I knew how people react, particularly people with whom you might be in business. It's very difficult for them to look at you as a long-term asset; in fact they all but write you off. And the other side of the coin is everyone who's a friend or even some who are only an acquaintance want to call and express their regrets that you have the problem, and all that really does is continue to remind you that you have the problem. It's nice to know they're concerned, but a card or email will suffice. I don't believe that commiserating helps, I think laughter helps. For those reasons, and although I was frank with my friends with whom I was in close contact, I asked Kat not to say anything anyone who might be connected in any way to the writing business. It was very hard for her, as many of her dearest and closest friends are fellow writers. In fact we had a couple visiting us and spending the night only two nights before we were to fly off. I consider them good friends, but they were in the writing business so I specifically asked Kat not to mention the problem to them. Besides, it's a much better time if everyone is mentally up and smiling (and better for your health), not down and moaning and dragging each other through health problems and hospital horror stories.

Immediately after they left we began packing for a week in Houston.

After an uneventful flight from Missoula to Denver to Houston, we checked into a hotel and had a Sunday of rest before appearing front and center at M. D. Anderson.

To say the least, it was a surprise.

Your cancer is your business and yours alone.

Like all diseases, it carries a certain stigma with it. If you're not comfortable in sharing the news of your diagnosis, then don't. I find that repeated calls from friends and family only serve to remind me that I have a problem. On the other hand, it's nice to know that you're loved and cared about.

17

I'M SOMEWHAT OF A CURMUDGEON WHEN IT comes to the path our society has taken, particularly when it comes to how counter people and service people relate to the public. I'd been serving people all my life in one form or another, often behind a counter, often banging on doors selling something. And I hate the way I see young people acting and being trained, or should I say, not being trained, to relate to the customer.

IN FACT I've been working on a training film called "Who's the Boss?" Employees from the kid behind the counter where you buy your hamburger to the receptionist where you buy your insurance to, yes, the average receptionist or nurse where you go to be treated have forgotten, or never been taught, who the boss is. When asked, they say their shift manager, their general manager, etc. Well trained people in all walks of business know who's the boss, and know, in the final analysis, no paychecks would be written were it not for the customer. The customer is the boss. There would be no employees, no managers, no CFO's or CEO's, no board of directors, and no stockholders...at least not for long, if there were no customers.

At M. D. Anderson Cancer Center, from the parking attendant (yes, there's valet parking), to the cafeteria cashier, to the doctor walking down the hall, you are greeted and, if you look confused, asked if they can be of help. Kat and I got separated in the hospital, and looking a little lost, two different times someone asked Kat if they could help and offered to loan her their cell phones since she'd forgotten hers. M. D. Anderson seemed to be in the 22nd century when it comes to quality care, and in the 19th century when it comes to courtesy and polite service.

If it can be a pleasure under the circumstance, it was a pleasure to be there.

I WAS DOUBLY SURPRISED, when sitting and waiting for an appointment, afraid to leave to get a cup of coffee or tea or I'd miss my call, when a cart arrived and the attendants announced, "free coffee or tea!" They had things you could buy too, but the intent of the cart was "customer" service. In this instance it was patient service, but in the final analysis, everyone in that waiting room was a "customer." And volunteers appeared regularly with a smile and a free cup.

I'LL TELL you how really big the place is in a moment, and even though you are in fact a number and a photograph, you are made to feel like you're part of the family. I was, to be truthful, astonished, as it was diametrically opposed to what I expected.

I HATE statistics because they can be so skewed, however, the American Cancer Society says that one in two of us will develop cancer in our lifetime. In

2009 there were some 1.5 million cancer patients in the U.S.; prostate being the leader among men and breast among women. Men tend to have more cancer than women. One in six men will develop prostate cancer, one in eight women breast cancer.

18

WE WERE CHECKED IN, GIVEN A NUMBER, AND scheduled to see a surgeon. Of course, the first course of business was a finger down the throat. Choke reflex was hyper, as usual, but I refrained from a well-placed knee. As it happened, Dr. Claymen, head and neck surgeon, my first contact with an M. D. Anderson physician, was frank, open, and very likable. Again, I had the fiber optic scope up the nose and down the throat and the conclusion of the exam was "no surgery." It seems the option in most head and neck centers is to avoid surgery at all costs as the recuperation from tongue surgery is long and hard, with the patient often having to relearn to both swallow and talk, if he can ever do either very effectively in his future. I was referred to the dentist, medical oncologist, and the radiologist. So far, I was on the same path as I had been in Montana. I wanted verification that the Montana docs were correct, and was getting it.

We later learned Dr. Claymen was not particularly happy with the CT scan I'd received, and scheduled me for another. The PET scan was fine, thank God, as it was fairly claustrophobic, at least as compared to the CT.

After the standard blood workup, my next appointment was with the dental staff. M. D. Anderson has it's own. It was good that we'd attacked the potential dental problem immediately. The dental staff complimented my Missoula, Montana treatment and the resultant pulling of the three molars. The good news was I was already two weeks into the healing process, and no radiation could begin until I was at least three weeks healed. We'd made a wise and propitious decision in attacking the teeth.

One of the first things that aimed me toward M. D. Anderson for treatment was the fitting of a mouth stint by the dental staff. The stint was to be a simple device that was fitted to your teeth, kept your mouth ¾ open, and if you used it properly kept your tongue forward and in one place—critical if the death rays were going to hit exactly the right spot. In addition, as good as my dental care was in Montana, I felt preparing for radiation was unusual for them, and SOP for the dental staff at Anderson. In addition to hitting the right spot, the stint helps avoid structures that will be damaged by radiation, particularly the saliva glands in the cheek and the soft pallet. When it comes to dealing with something that might—will —effect you for the rest of your life, such as saliva gland function, taste bud function, and blood supply to a critical continually functioning structure such as the jaw, you want someone well practiced. That said, I was very proud of my home-town dental team.

After dental finished my exam and concluded I needed no additional work, I was off to see the medical oncologist, the chemo lady. Dr. Sabichi was a very attractive well-spoken woman who carefully explained my chemo options, but unlike Montana said it appeared I would need minimal chemo ther-apy, only a chemical solution that would make the cancer more susceptible to the radiation. And even that could be questionable.

Next, I was to see the radiologist. Dr. Gunn was properly named, having to be the one who "shot" me with the death rays. He was likable and wore cowboy boots—which shouldn't have been a surprise to me in

Houston. Having all my life thought cowboy boots the most manly of foot ware, and having a half-dozen pairs myself, I warmed to him immediately. He explained the process of radiation and it's after effects, which I already knew fairly well. Of course, again it was both the fingers down the throat and the scope up the nose and down the throat.

He also informed me of the coming meeting of all the docs involved to review my case, who'd examine me for what I hoped was one last time, and arrive at a consensus as to my treatment.

While awaiting that meeting, I had another CT scan.

Kat had been at my side during this whole process, and I honestly think it was harder on her than on me. Even though I actually had the needles, fingers, scopes, and infernal machines, she had to watch and listen to me retch, and I think watching may in many instances be worse than the actuality. But then she's an empathetic lady.

We had a few days to kill. We had come to the conclusion that M. D. Anderson was the place to be for the next two months, so rather than suffer the cost and constriction of a hotel room, we looked for an apartment. Because of the huge medical community in the city, there are a number of short term rentals available. For just over a hundred dollars a day (the same price as a small hotel room near the hospital) we found a two bedroom, two bath, apartment overlooking a pool and a mere one hundred feet from the complex's gymnasium. I had visions of being able to continue to work, write, while undergoing treatment, and Kat had deadlines to fulfill, so the space for office equipment was imperative. We were more than satisfied with the apartment, but could not commit until we knew exactly when we were to return, and that decision would follow the "consensus of treatment" meeting.

That meeting consisted of four docs, again with the fingers down the throat and the fiber optic scope, only this time the results were on a monitor the size of our home TV. I was facing away so I didn't get a look at the monster causing me to be here in Houston and not back in Montana tending my garden and getting ready for hunting season.

DON'T SMOKE.

19

I WAS VERY, VERY PLEASED WITH THE conclusion of the "consensus meeting," as the docs decided I did not need chemo.

Interestingly, every step of the way since I first discovered the knot in my neck, and since it grew (post fine needle biop) to about three centimeters in length and two in width, it had not changed in size. No growth. I have no way of proving that my juicing and use of the Ojibwa medicine man's concoction had any effect on this, but cancer grows, at times voraciously, and mine had not, at least not in a way that was perceptive to me.

Maybe, just maybe, I'd saved myself from the debilitating and sickening poisoning of the body that is chemotherapy by juicing and using the tea? No chemo was going to make things easier to bare. Not that I thought the radiation was going to be a walk in the park, I knew better as they were going to burn out the knot in my neck and the tumor on the back of my tongue. There may be spots on the body where a deep burn might be more painful, but it's hard to imagine where.

I say "on the back of my tongue" rather than "in the back of my tongue," because one of the other conclusions of the docs meeting was that the tumor was not deeply ingrained in the muscle that is the tongue.

Kat and I packed up, with some new enthusiasm, and flew back to Montana.

We weren't sure exactly when our next appointment would be, but were advised to return within a week, and that week would include a 2013 mile drive.

We arrived at the Missoula air terminal just before midnight on a Saturday, and made the twenty-eight mile drive home. I can't tell you how happy we were to be back in Montana, even for a very short time. I was particularly happy because I felt, for the first time, confident that I was going to beat this monster. The black cloud of my good friend's one month survival had been hanging over my head, but my tumor hadn't seemed to have grown in the six weeks or more since I'd discovered it, and I had a path I was on to exorcise it from my body. I felt strong, and more so because I had direction.

We're fairly used to "leaving" home for some length of time as for the last five years we've been chickening out on the Montana winters and relocating to our second home in California (considered by us to be an investment more than "home") for four months, and for the last couple of years for the month of August as well. So it's been five months in California and seven months in Montana, not counting travel time to several writing conferences and research trips each year. So, packing up for some extended time was not new to us.

Kat was working under a deadline, and both of us have always prided ourselves on making our deadlines in an industry, publishing, that's somewhat famous for missing contractual obligations. That would mean that she had to continue writing even though we had this small matter of a cancer to deal with. And that would mean we had to have computers and printers and research materials and myriad office paraphernalia as well as clothes and personal items to last a couple of months. In the case of the California house we have left items there that we didn't have to haul back and forth; we had nothing in Houston, other than one file box we'd left knowing we were returning.

To show how much confidence I'd developed: I'd ordered some golf clubs just before discovering the cancer, and, concerned with the fact I'd have no need of golf clubs, or food, water, or air, in the near future, I'd cancelled the order. I reaffirmed it. It made me feel better and gave me a boost in confidence. While I was worrying about the yard and horses, etc., Kat was confirming our apartment rental and getting ready to be away from her office (which is in the Montana house as is mine) and all the research materials she has readily at hand in our offices and library.

We decided not to tarry. We'd attacked this problem from the onset and decided we'd continue to charge forward. We were packed and on the road by Wednesday morning. The car was packed, and I mean that in the literal sense of the word.

Luckily, my oldest son had remodeled the old farm house on the property we have in Montana, so he and his two sons, two of our six grandchildren, live only a couple of hundred yards away, and I could depend upon them to pick up on any loose ends I had left in closing up the house.

Spending the first night in Sheridan was a pleasure for us, as we appreciate all things western and Sheridan, Wyoming is the shining example of a classic western town. Kat and I have both written novels set in the west, and over half my novels are, in fact, westerns. We're both students of the old west, and members of Western Writers of America as well as other professional writer's groups. And I love the drive there and on to Denver as the highway is lined with deer, elk, and antelope, and all the smaller birds and animals that make the Pacific Northwest and the Rocky Mountains such a pleasure.

The next night was spent on the southeast side of Denver, where we met up with old friends and enjoyed a good supper. The following night was spent on the south side of Oklahoma City.

We rolled into our new, if temporary, home in Houston to find the key under the mat.

Cancer is not a death sentence. The Mayo Clinic says that 98 out of every hundred men with prostate cancer are alive in five years. No matter what statistics say, take a hard look at those being reported upon. In my case, with throat cancer, almost all cases involved men who smoked heavily and drank heavily. I have never smoked and am a 6 oz of red wine a night guy, with my supper. I immediately assumed I was a lot more healthy than the average throat cancer victim. A little positive thinking goes a long way. Attitude is everything. I'm going to repeat that because I think it's so important:

ATTITUDE IS EVERYTHING!

20

The University of Texas M. D. Anderson Cancer Center inspires awe. Not just because of its size with over 17,000 employees and 1,300 volunteers, but because of its permeating attitude. One would think, as I mentioned before, that you would be merely a number when you're among the almost 100,000 patients treated each year; when you wander among, if I counted properly, the eleven multi-story buildings on the "main campus." In almost every publication from the Anderson, and there are a plethora, the word compassion is used, and it's not merely given lip service by the staff, it seems to saturate the organization. But I'll let the man where the buck stops speak for the Anderson.

This from a letter introducing a booklet: At Your Service: Handbook for Patients.

Welcome to The University of Texas M. D. Anderson Cancer Center. You have come to a very special place, a center of excellence with a rich history. For more than 60 years, M. D. Anderson has been a worldwide leader in cancer patient care, research, education, and prevention.

At M. D. Anderson, you will find a health care team dedicated to providing you with the best possible care. On your team are specialists from every field related to the diagnosis and treatment of cancer. These experts will combine their knowledge and skills to develop a treatment plan specifically for you.

You, too, are an important member of your health care team. Your understanding and cooperation are vital ingredients in your care. We hope you will read this booklet carefully and keep it for future reference. And, whenever you have questions, please ask a member of your team for help.

We are committed to providing you with the service, quality of care and compassion you and your family expect. At M. D. Anderson, the patient always comes first.

John Mendelsohn, M. D.

President

Upon first seeing this impressive facility I couldn't help but wonder who M. D. Anderson was or might have been. I presumed, since Houston is the epicenter of oil fortunes in the United States, that he was an oilman who was instrumental in the creation and endowment of the institution. Coming from an oil rich county in California, it was a somewhat natural assumption. However, Kern County, California is also one of the great agricultural counties in the United States, and cotton is, or was for many years, considered king. As Anderson, Clayton and Company had operations there, I should not have been surprised, when upon reading Making Cancer History, by James S. Olson, professor of history at Sam Houston State University, that it was cotton, not oil, that brought the Anderson name to the hospital.

By the time Monroe D. Anderson, known as Mon to his friends and relatives, passed away in 1939 he had amassed a fortune of nineteen million dollars, and that's when a million was a million. He funded the M. D. Anderson Foundation for the "establishment, support and maintenance of hospitals, homes and institutions for the care of the sick," in addition to the promotion of "health, science, education, and advancement and diffusion of understanding among the people."

One of the partners, John Freeman, of the law firm entrusted with the estate often dined with Houston physician Ernst W. Bertner, who was active with the American Society for the Control of Cancer. With the support of Arthur Cato, a Texas politician, in 1941 the Texas legislature appropriated a half million dollars to fund a state cancer hospital to be affiliated with the University of Texas. After much competition, Houston was selected as a location for the hospital, encouraged by the offer of the Anderson Foundation to match the half million, should the hospital be located in Houston. Both Freeman and Bertner were instrumental in that offer, and out politic'd many of the states best politicians.

The foundation quickly purchased a six acre estate, complete with large house, barns, and outbuildings, and gave the property to the hospital. Bertner became the interim director, and even with the war going on, materials were obtained to remodel the house into a clinic and the barns and outbuildings into laboratories and necessary facilities.

And the University of Texas M. D. Anderson Cancer Center was born and in 1942 was named the

M. D. Anderson Hospital for Cancer Research of the University of Texas. It was March of 1944 before the hospital accepted it's first patient. That same year Lee Clark, a brilliant surgeon, took over as director of the hospital.

I hope that somewhere from a very comfortable seat on a cloud, Mon Anderson is gazing down at what his hard work and thrift brought to Houston, and the world.

I intend to discover the cause of cancer and build the greatest cancer hospital in the world.

R. Lee Clark, 1946

21

It was time to be treated for squamous head and neck cancer.

I had picked up my mouth stint and tried it in the dentist's presence. It seemed to fit fine. The device is fitted to your teeth and has a plate at the bottom so you can slip your tongue under, somewhat protecting it and keeping it out of the direct line of the death rays. But more importantly, it keeps your tongue in exactly the right position so the target is consistently in the same place.

The generic name of Valium is Diazepam and my doctors in Missoula had kindly give me a prescription for 5 mg tablets after I confessed my severe claustrophobia. I was advised that taking one an hour before treatment would suffice. And it got me thorough my PET scan. But Kat was convinced that it had some kind of opposite effect on me, and I'd actually gotten more hyper after I got up from the table. So in preparation for my actual treatments, the docs in Houston prescribed Lorazepam.

I'd taken only one of the 1 mg tablets an hour before my first treatment was scheduled.

I'd like to say I was relaxed when walking into that first treatment wherein I'd be pegged down to a cold stainless steel table under a fifteen foot by ten foot monster-praying-mantis of a machine, with its two foot round, one-eyed, flat face ominously staring down from less than a foot away, but I'd be lying.

I kicked off my shoes and stripped away my shirt, as requested, and the attendant, Chuck, brought me my mouth stint. It immediately chocked me when I tried to fit it in place, in fact gagged me. Now, was this a psychosomatic response to keep me from having to be strapped down? I don't know, but I rebelled and said I'd have to go back to dental to have the stint "shaved down."

Receiving no argument from the slightly frustrated but very compassionate death ray crew, I escaped. It was very hard to go back into that waiting room and tell my wife I'd failed my first test under fire. But I had. I could see in her eyes that she had her doubts that I'd ever climb under the monster. She'd seen me climb many a stair rather than get in an elevator.

We headed up ten floors or so to the dental department and waited for Dr. Chambers, who was very accommodating. They probably shaved 1/8" off the inch and one half depth, behind the teeth, where the stint penetrated deep into my mouth.

The next day I appeared front and center at radiation, only this time I'd prescribed my own dose of Lorazepam, taking two and a half of those small 1 mg tablets, and I was bouncing off the walls. Even at that, being pegged down to the machine, your head and face completely covered and your upper body pinned to below the shoulders was traumatic.

There are maybe eight pegs that are turned into receptors on the table that hold you in place, so you can't move a millimeter. As each peg was turned, sucking the mask down, I wondered just how tight this mask was to be, and could I possibly escape on my own if necessary? To keep you from moving a millimeter, you can only imagine how tight the mask was.

I felt as if I'd been shrink-wrapped to the table.

Laser lights from the ceiling are aligned with marks placed on your mask and body (ink lines that stay during treatment), and their alignment is carefully attended to by the two actually giving the treatment, Chuck and Wie in my case. The care and compassion of these two was integral to my comfort. The first treatment is, of course, all new, and the lights, sounds, and motions of the room and equipment, particularly when all you can do is cut your eyes, seems amplified.

I had gone through radiation before with my prostate cancer, so I knew there would be no feeling from the actual rays penetrating your body, and there was none.

The first treatment is rather long because they are taking x-rays as well, with the same machine, to make sure they are hitting the target, and, as efficiently as possible, avoiding the other major structures in your neck.

With the help of the Lorazepam, I made it through the thirty minutes or so of being pegged down without making any attempt to rip myself from the table and run screaming from the hospital. In fact, when Chuck quickly appeared to release me, I had a certain sense of satisfaction that I'd slain the dragon...still I was not eager to face him again.

Of course, I was still bouncing off the walls, and, like a pint of whiskey consumed in a bar full of beautiful women, two and a half milligrams of Lorazepam make you feel 6' 6" and 250 fifty pounds of pure muscle. So I'd been tough enough to take on the monster.

Now the target is to cut down the dose so I'm not ka ka faced all the time.

Cancer treatment is constantly improving. The overall five year cancer survival rate went up from 49.3 percent in 1976 to 53.9 percent in 1990. All you've got to do to beat the odds is to be one of those who fall in the 53.9 percentile. Nothing to it.

Not only is better treatment a part of that increased survival rate, but early detection is a large part. Be proactive about your health!

22

Treatment two was only slightly easier, but one of the nice asides of waiting to be treated is the waiting room, full of nice folks with the same or worse problems than your own, and their relatives, friends, and supporters. I was surprised to meet a nice gentleman and his lady friend from Kalispell, not far north of where we live. He'd traveled a couple of hundred miles more than we did to get treated at the Anderson, and he was a retired physician. It gave me another boost of confidence that I'd chosen correctly.

I was equally impressed with another lovely lady who had brain cancer and was shaved bald under her cowboy hat and above her hoop earrings. At about my same age, she managed to look as if she'd stepped out of Vogue, rather than stepping into a treatment room.

You rapidly become a student of those who've had more treatments than you and a mentor to those with fewer. Topics of conversation are, "what are you eating?" and "what are you doing for the burns?" In addition to the niceties of family and daily life while in a strange city reporting to the hospital every weekday.

Those in the waiting room began to seem like old friends as the treatments moved on.

In addition to the treatments we had a consult with Dr. Gunn each Wednesday and one more consult with Dr. Sabichi, the medical oncologist, who again confirmed that I didn't need chemo. I also had additional blood work done before seeing her so she could check my meds.

During the first two weeks I cut my dose of happy pills down until I was free of them. I didn't begin feeling any soreness until about treatment number eight, then with number ten it began to really affect my ability to swallow and my taste was almost totally gone.

One of the things that helped distract me was music. I loaded my iPod up with all the great music I love and took my little iPod boom box into the treatment room, turned it up as loud as they'd allow, and let good friends Willy, Santana, Celine, Whitney, etc. keep me company. The machine is relatively quiet, with a little gear noise and a buzz when it's actually zapping you, so the music can easily over rule, or at least compete with that. Stimulus of the ears is the best entertainment, for there's little to see, and as it pays to keep your eyes shut, particularly when the one-eyed monster is directly in your face only nine inches away.

You can't imagine how unattractive food becomes when you lose your sense of taste. And that from a guy who's always been a foody. I probably own a hundred cookbooks and Kat and I make good restaurants a hobby. For the past couple of years I have been working on a TV show The Kitchen at Wolfpack Ranch (and now have a cooking/kitchen website I'd love to have you visit: wolfpackranch.-com), which I'd submitted to PBS, the Outdoor Channel, and Rural TV. I've had a lot of interest and many nice compliments on the layout and style of the show, and many suggestions regarding improving the technical aspects, i.e. sound, lighting, editing. The fact is I tried to find professional help in Montana, but it's almost impossible. I decided to learn the craft of film making myself and acquired a couple of Mac computers, Final Cut Studio, lights, and sound equipment. Obviously I was still not quite up to speed with them, but learned a whole lot. All that came to a screaming halt with a tumor on the back of my tongue, and more so when I began to lose my taste buds. Que sara.

Sometimes it takes great courage to take the first step of a thousand mile journey. Then, to your surprise, every step thereafter becomes easier and easier.

23

I have joined the now generation and both have a website for my writing, www.ljmartin.com, and one for my cooking, www.wolfpackranch.com; and I developed Kat's original website,

www.katbooks.com

It's now well maintained by a very capable executive assistant who is multi-talented. I've posted a number of both cooking and how-to-get-published videos to YouTube.com with the user name ljmartin-wolfpack.

Actually, being a curious devil, I started writing websites twenty years ago when one was still writing HTML by hand, after going to a class with this new business on the block, the Internet Service Provider.

Additions to the current websites will have to wait a while.

I'm told, should I whip the disease, my taste buds will return (they have, 100% I'd guess). One doc says three months post treatment; one says six. Will the buds ever be the same? I have no idea. I can't imagine a situation where I can't write, but where I can't cook? Why cook if you can't taste? How can you develop recipes if you can't taste?

But I have reinvented myself several times over the years, from architectural draftsman, to water company manager, to real estate salesman, to contractor, to appraiser, to writer, to aspiring TV cook, so maybe another reinvention will be in order... God willing and the creek don't rise. I always did want to try and make some documentaries. Along those career paths, I was a cook both by vocation and avocation, and a photographer by avocation since I carried a 4" x 5" Speed Graphic as the junior high photographer.

After a latter half of a lifetime watching my weight by weighing every day and making sure I don't exceed one eighty five (now 176), the challenge now becomes not losing weight, keeping up the caloric intake and particularly the protein intake when you can't taste what you're eating. Eating is suddenly an unpleasant chore rather than a joy. My routine has become: a Boost ® drink with grams of protein first thing in the morning; a shake made in the blender using a banana, a peach or other fruit, some protein powder (27 grams worth), and either milk or soy milk. An Odwala ® drink—the monster protein variety with 33 grams of protein, and maybe another shake in the evening. The object is to get 80 grams of protein a day as it seems the radiology eats muscle, and to keep up your caloric intake. Kat says I need 2,500 calories a day, but I can't force near that much down. Herein lies another problem: cancer loves glucose (sugar) and loves mucus. Milk products produce mucus. Yet you have to eat, and when sugar is about all you can taste, but barely even that....

One of my favorite pieces of country wisdom is one
I've repeated to myself over and over:
I cried about having no shoes...until I met a man with
no feet.

24

AN OLD FRIEND OF MINE FROM MY HOME TOWN of Bakersfield arrived here in Houston with his wife, and with the same problem as mine, so I became somewhat of a mentor. It gave me some distraction, as did my cameras and my computer. I'm in the middle of writing a thriller, a suspense (see my now 50 books on Amazon, search L. J. Martin), and this journal, and for the first time in years have bought some computer games to take up the time I'd not be spending in the garden or yard or on the golf course near home. The docs promptly informed me I was to stay out of the sun, so there went the golf. I still could pull out my putter and use the carpet for a green.

I finished my thirteenth treatment the Friday before the Labor Day holiday, so it'll be next

Tuesday that I'll enjoy my fifteenth—half way through. The next day I'll have a double session, a treatment in the morning and one in the afternoon, to make up for the techs getting Labor Day off. That should be extra fun.

It's now a lot of work to swallow. My saliva is cut way down, as I expected, however the mucus in my throat also seems to have increased. I imagine that's a reaction of my body against the radiation burns. So you still are compelled to swallow every few minutes.

I've had strep throat before, and if you've had it you know what a sore throat is all about. The fourteen treatments gradually built up the sore throat until it's almost that bad, as well as has caused some skin reddening and irritation down to a level about three inches below the base of the neck both front and back.

When you have very little saliva, a dead mouth taste-wise, and a burned knot on the base of your tongue so far back you can't run an index finger down to touch it, you wake up in the night thinking a Houston-sized super cockroach has crawled into your gaping mouth and burrowed into the base of your tongue. That, alone, is enough to kill your appetite.

The docs advise you to rinse your mouth and gargle with a baking soda-water solution, and I've been faithfully doing so four or five times a day. It supposedly helps to keep the mouth sores at bay, and so far is successful. A couple of places feel like I've bitten my tongue, which I haven't done, but at least the sore spots are not open and ulcerated. I've been using an external 99% Aloe liquid to treat the redness (burns) and an internal Aloe solution to rinse the mouth, gargle, and swallow. Our solution and it works well. They also advise you to exercise your jaw as the radiation takes away muscle and limits movement. My first dentist in Missoula advised me of this and gave me a marked plastic stick to show how far my mouth opened prior to treatment. I've gauged that every day to make sure I was staying limber in the jaw department. God knows I'd hate to be limited in flapping my jaw, although many friends and family might be happy for the condition.

They've also given me a prescription, a mouth rinse made especially in the M. D. Anderson pharmacy, to deaden the pain.

Maybe it's time to give it a try.

Sleep is a critical component of any healing process, and to my way of thinking in fighting any illness, including cancer. Of course, when you've been told you have cancer, it's only normal that it keeps you awake nights. And I, for one, hate sleeping pills. The best solution is exercise and natural sleep inducers such as melatonin in good old milk...warm milk. Of course there's a theory that cancer loves mucus and milk produces mucus. This is typical of the dilemmas you face when trying to figure out what the hell to do to help your body fighting this ugly invader.

I believe it was Ford who said "if you believe you can, or can't, your right."

25

I MAY BE A HARDHEAD, BUT I'VE MANAGED TO stay off the pain medicine.

Today may kick me over to rinsing my mouth with the M. D. Anderson's witchdoctor's brew, especially made for radiation sores in the mouth. Today may be the day because I have two treatments scheduled and a doc appointment. They schedule the treatments at least six hours apart, so my first is at 9:30 AM and second at 3:30 PM.

The best laid plans of mice and men...the first treatment didn't come off until 10:30 and the doc's appointment is 1:30 so we go home to work for a couple of hours.

The knot in my neck has not receded as we hoped it would and we question the doc regarding that. It concerns us, needless to say. He explains that the knot may stay the same size even if the cells are dead, however he agrees to do another CT scan, which will be compared to the first, to make sure it's not larger. One can always conclude, after watching too many horror movies, that the cancer is actually feeding on the death rays.

So we return in the afternoon for a CT scan, which is performed with the mask on. It's only a few minutes as they only scan from nose to the base of the neck. We'll bug the doc for the results tomorrow.

Then it's back downstairs to the thick-walled dungeon to the treatment department, where we're finally seen about 4:30 as the last treatment of the day. Chuck is the last of the Mohicans and does the treatment himself. As always, I'm impressed by his upbeat manner even though he's having to work alone and I'm keeping him late.

It seems there is some adjustment necessary to the path of the death rays, so maybe our questioning the size of the tumor in the neck has had some positive effect.

As always, there's no feeling involved in the treatment, other than being shrink-wrapped to the table for a quarter of an hour. But I can't help but think that this rapid repetition of the treatment will add to the burns on the skin and in the mouth.

I've gotten in the habit of taking my Aloe with me and as soon as we're in the car, I apply it to the skin, which is beginning to prickle. I'll apply it three or four more times before I hit the sack.

The treatments have become rote, which I'm sure is helpful to the crew. As soon as I enter the room with the monster death ray machine, I set up my boom box, peel off my shoes and shirt, slip the stint in my mouth, and assume the position on the table, on my back. As I mentioned much earlier, there's a plastic formed neck brace attached to the tabletop which throws your head back. If you position yourself on the table so your neck and head fits exactly into the rest, you're very close to the treatment position. A foam rubber rest is fitted under your knees and a footboard, with ropes and wraps that fit around your wrists, is positioned. This is so you can push with your feet and pull your shoulders down. You would think this confining, as if our hands are being tied down, but you're in complete control and if you let up pressure on the board, you can remove the wraps from your wrist. In fact, they instruct you to raise your knees if you're having a problem, such as choking, and they'll turn off the machine and hustle to your aid. The table is raised to about counter height. Then the mask is fitted and secured to the table. The lights are lowered so the laser lights are easily seen and aligned. Usually there are two attendants in the room who then use the lasers to make sure the ink marks on your body are exact, and I mean exact. They then position your body so lasers hit marks. The table itself is adjustable, electrically and mechanically, to the millimeter, both up, down, left, right, back, and forward. When both attendants are happy with your location, the overhead lights are switched back on and they leave the room.

The two foot circular head of the machine moves from a position very low and out of sight to the left or right depending upon the operator, in a circular motion on a vertical plane from position to position until it's passed directly over your face at about nine inches away, to a position low on the other side. Making about nine stops along the way. This is the time when your friends Willy, Dion, and Alabama are the only ones in the room with you, and you're glad to have them as company.

When the call comes over the intercom, "You can raise your knees now," you're done with treatment. They hustle into the room and free you from the mask. They lower the table and you're ready, really ready, to escape. You pack up your stuff, don shoes and shirt, and you're out of there.

Courage is not always a roar, sometimes it creeps in
on cat paws and whispers,
"tomorrow will be better."

26

THIS AFTERNOON, AFTER MY 17TH TREATMENT, my cell phone rang and it was Dr. Gunn, who'd looked at the CT scan and announced that, yes, as Kat and I suspected, the tumor had grown.

You are taken aback, even if it's your own suspicions confirmed.

Dr. Gunn explained that cystic tumors such as mine become liquefied during treatment, and it is not uncommon for them to grow, or swell, somewhat. Mine, he said, was only a half-centimeter longer, but was 30% greater in volume. He proposed to do two extra treatments, only to the neck tumor and not to the tongue tumor. This means that tomorrow—which was to be an unusual day none-the-less as one machine was being worked on and they were doubling patients on another—I was to report at 8:00 AM rather than 10:30; now I'd be reporting at 8:00 AM for a normal treatment and again after 2:00 PM for a second treatment. The same would hold for Monday, two treatments.

These special treatments will be different than the norm in that they are electron beam radiotherapy. I understand the beam is limited as to the depth it penetrates, so it's ideal for a tumor resting just under the skin.

Dr. Gunn was in the treatment room when I arrived and he and the attendant, Mary, spent a lot of time setting up the machine. I thought this was only going to take a very few minutes so I didn't set up my iPod, and eventually wished I had. As it happened it took about the same time as a regular treatment. More ink marks, this time, only around the neck tumor to delineate it. Wherein they used the CT scan and computer to set up the regular treatments, they did this one manually.

Awaking the next morning, Saturday, I felt some rawness for the first time on the margins of the neck tumor, so I guess this electron beam hits pretty hard.

So far I'm still able to swallow with little real problem so that's not the primary problem in keeping the weight up, it's the lack of taste. You'd think you'd become inured to eating without taste, and maybe I will, but not yet. I'm trying to keep a water bottle in hand or on the desk or on the coffee table in front of the TV at all times, to encourage me to stay hydrated, and have been pretty successful so far. It's harder with the Boost ® or Odwalla ® but I'm still knocking down about 80 grams of protein a day, but only 1,000 calories or so. Not enough. My weight's down from 185 to 171 as of last Wednesday and I'll be surprised if it doesn't fall off to 165 before this is over, maybe lower as even when the radiation is finished, I'll still be unable to taste for six months. I graduated high school at about 155, so I guess I can fall that low, and I guess if I have to have all my suits tailored, and that's the worst result from having throat cancer, I'll be one of the luckiest guys ever to prowl the halls of M. D. Anderson.

Speaking of that, when I left the hospital yesterday, seeing a lot of folks in wheelchairs from their cancer and more so from their chemo and radiation treatment, I felt very fortunate. I had to laugh and point out to Kat that it's strange to have throat cancer and feel fortunate, then I remembered one of my favorite sayings: I cried about having no shoes until I met a man with no feet.

We're off today to Whole Foods, the health food market, to see if we can find a drink that is healthful, full of protein, and full of calories, but with much less sugar than those I've been using.

Not trying is the same as failing.

27

I'VE NOW COMPLETED FIVE WEEKS OF RADIATION, 24 regular treatments plus two electron beam treatments. I'm still off the serious pain medication, but my throat is sore and I don't know if I'll make it through another week without. I am dropping three to four Advil ®, particularly at night as it seems to help me sleep.

I've got quite a bit of mucus in my throat, which I presume is a natural reaction of your body against the burns. It's hard to swallow, but I'm still managing to get down a couple of Boost ® and an Odwalla ® everyday, as well as a couple of cups of tea and a little Gatorade ®. Nothing tastes like anything, but the Boost ® and Odwalla ® are very smooth, and the Gatorade ® is refreshing. Anything hot or cold hurts, so I let the cold stuff warm up and take the tea, and a Boost ® in the morning—substituting for a hot chocolate, but only lukewarm.

My tongue feels as if I've both burned and bitten it, and the back of my throat feels as if I'm belching ashes. I know that's my imagination, but it's not much fun. Then I didn't expect much fun when I came here.

You get to be on a first name basis with the crew in both the docs office and the dungeon where you get zapped. After I finished my last treatment, I couldn't help but say to Chuck how much I appreciate his and Wie's attitude, and how much I respected how they made the treatments as comfortable as possible, and he had an interesting reply. One that impressed me even more than the president's letter that I quoted earlier. Chuck's reply was, "If you're in it for the money, you don't last long around here."

I found that poignant and touching, and it well represented the attitude of everyone I came across at M. D. Anderson.

In addition to being one of the great treatment hospitals, M. D. Anderson is a teaching hospital and research institution. Of the ninety thousand plus patients treated each year, thirty thousand are new, and nearly thirteen thousand participated in clinical trials exploring novel treatments, the largest such program in the nation.

Last year there were over one thousand active clinical research protocols underway.

In addition, almost a million outpatient clinic visits, treatments, and procedures are performed, and, believe it or not, almost ten million pathology/lab medicine procedures are performed.

I can testify to only one example of the "lab" procedures and that's blood work. You enter a waiting room that must be seventy-five feet square and sign in. In minutes you're called, usually one of five or so read off at the same time, and go into get your blood drawn. Your card is checked, verifying your bar code and patient number, and you're out of there in a very few minutes. There must be at least ten phlebotomists at work drawing blood. And all of them with a smile on their faces.

It's truly an amazing place.

While the rest of the country is crying about health care, which seems strange to me as all one has to do is walk into any hospital to be cared for—it's the law—M. D. Anderson provided Two Hundred Eight Million Seven Hundred Thousand Dollars in unsponsored charity care to Texans with cancer in 2008.

I can't help but believe that Mon Anderson, perched on his cloud, is very, very proud, as he should be.

Our national symbol is the bald eagle. It soars far and wide looking for sustenance and solutions. The oyster rests awaiting the solution to come to him. Be an eagle, not an oyster; seek and ye shall find.

28

THE HOSPITAL GENERATED OVER TWO AND A half billion dollars in revenue in 2008. Patients accounted for 78.3% of that. Grants, contracts, and philanthropy kicked in another 13.6%. The State of Texas came through with 6.1%, and the small balance was other income and auxiliary enterprises.

In addition to excellent patient care, six thousand physicians, scientists, nurses, and allied health professionals were involved in educational programs at the hospital, which awards bachelor's degrees in seven health disciplines. It also awards M.S. and Ph.D. degrees at the University of Texas School of Biomedical Sciences.

When I was treated by the electron beam machine, two medical students observed the set up of the procedure, and at least twice students have been observing when I received my normal week day treatments.

In addition to over seventeen thousand employees and almost fifteen hundred volunteers, M. D. Anderson has a faculty of almost fifteen hundred. The North Campus, where I was treated, consists of the Main Building, Alkek Hospital, Bates-Freeman Building, Clark Clinic, Gimbel Building, Jones Research Building, LeMaistre Clinic, Love Clinic, and the Lutheran Hospital Pavilion.

Nearby are the Cancer Prevention Building, Clinical Research Building, Faculty Center, Jones Rotary House International (where patients can be housed), Mays Clinic, Mitchell Basic Sciences Research Building, and the Pickens Academic Tower.

In addition to all this, there's the South Campus with another five buildings, as well as clinical care centers in other locations.

The hospital is affiliated with an extensive physicians network, with twenty sister institution relationships in Europe, the Middle East, Asia, and North and South America.

And the M. D. Anderson is part of a larger Texas Medical Center complex of 47 institutions which include 13 hospitals, 19 academic institutions, and 15 support services organizations. The 11 diploma or degree granting educational institutions are made up of schools of dentistry, public health, pharmacy, four nursing schools, and two medical schools.

It seems, in Houston, there's a hospital or medical institution every time your turn a corner.

As I received my 25th treatment this morning, a medical student was in attendance.

If 29.6 million current gross square feet of building doesn't impress you, maybe the seven billion in planned projects, including new hospitals, clinics, research and other office space by the Texas Medical Center will...it's certainly impressed me. It's said to equal the 13th largest business district in the United States.

When I came here I had no idea the extent of the investment in medical facilities in and around the University of Texas M. D. Anderson Cancer Center.

All I knew is that I was one guy with a cancer that scared the hell of out of him, and that he wanted to be rid of.

As Yogi said, "when you come to a fork in the road, take it." You are always one choice away from changing your life.

29

Today is my 27th and 28th treatment—it's a twofer day, in addition to my usual Wednesday visit to the Dr. Gunn, my radiation oncologist. I will be weighed and have my blood pressure taken, both sitting then a minute later standing. This is a way to check and see how dehydrated you might be. If your pressure maintains when standing, then you have little or no dehydration. If it falls, which it did the last time I had it taken, from 140 down to 120 on the top end, then you're dehydrated. Seems when throats get real sore folks stop swallowing, even water. Last week I passed the dehydration test, this week I was a little dehydrated. The good news was Dr. Gunn had mentioned taking a look with the dreaded fiber optic device that would be run up my nose and into my throat, then decided he could see enough just scoping down my throat. I dodged that bullet.

My neck is red as a crawdad, particularly on the tumor. The color is actually a little more deep plum than red. It doesn't hurt that badly, unless you rub it, which we do about five times a day with aloe. The aloe seems to be working as my necks in much better shape than some of those in the waiting room who are about the same stage of treatment.

I'm still rinsing my mouth several times a day with a water/baking soda mix, and so far I have no open sores in my mouth. The back of my throat feels like a chunk of busted concrete has taken up residence there, and there are visible blister-like formations, much whiter than the rosy red a mouth should be, on the sides of my tongue and the back of my throat. My uvula, the dangly thing in the back of your throat, is almost totally white. I presume, totally blistered.

Open questioning my new friend Chuck, the attendant at the death ray machine, informs me that what I'm feeling is more than likely esophagitis.

Esophagitis is an inflammation of the esophagus, the food tube. It's sensitive to radiation and becomes inflamed and sore during treatment. This explains a good portion of the "lump of concrete" I feel in the back of my throat and the pain upon attempting to swallow. I'm told, both by my physicians and the internet that these symptoms will reside within three weeks of completing treatment. I wonder what I'll weigh in a month?

In addition, I've developed mucositis, which is an inflammation of the lining of the mouth and gums. My gums now feel rough to the touch. Mucositis is a thickening of your saliva, which actually feels stringy. And there's less of it, which results in dry-mouth.

Both of these conditions make eating uncomfortable if not impossible. Where eating was always an abject pleasure, it's now an irritation and discomforting interruption.

You must continue to dwell on the consequence of not undergoing treatment, in order to push you through the treatment and resulting discomfort.

I'm very tired in the afternoon, and this day, only three days from the end, I have to go back for my 2nd shot of death rays for the day—this is my own fault as I chickened out the first day and they like to end treatments on a Friday, which, thank God, is day after tomorrow.

We've begun messing around packing, getting

ready to head back to Montana. I'm told we'll have to come back in 6 to 10 weeks for a follow up, a period which I'm sure will be full of anxiety as you'll be wondering if this torture-treatment really worked.

The good news is I'll be busy in Montana.

"The difference between a successful person and others is not a lack of strength, not a lack of knowledge, but rather a lack of will."
--Vince Lombardi

30

It's been a long road from discovering this small lump on my neck to this last day of treatment. During the thirty days of actually sitting in the waiting room, we've got to rejoice many times with folks who got to "ring the bell," which is a rite of passage for those who've finished radiation. Mounted on the wall in a hallway is ship's bell, much like the one I still have mounted over my bar at home, a remembrance of a time I owned a boat big enough to have a ship's bell mounted on her main mast. Today's my day to "ring the bell."

As I've mentioned, you develop some real friendships with patients and their friends and relatives in the waiting room. There is no question everyone there has something in common, and certainly a basis for conversation. I hope to see these folks again, under much happier circumstance.

The only time since I've been taking treatments, my iPod failed me, however, Chuck had a great album on and I enjoyed it as much or more than listening to the same old songs on my machine.

It was almost strange as I sat myself on the table then lay in place, with my head in the plastic receptacle. For the first time, I was perfectly aligned and they didn't have to push, pull, tug, or cajole my body into exactly the right position for treatment. It was as if I was finally well practiced. I guess the last of 32 treatments "getting it right" was better than never getting it right.

Both Chuck and Wie seemed truly pleased that I had gotten through the treatments as well as I had. I had never "raised my knees" to stop treatment once it had begun, and was secretly proud of that, as many times I felt as if I was going to choke, and have to panic and raise my knees to signal them to run into the room. But I overcame it.

Upon releasing me from the table, Chuck informed me that I was a good a patient as they'd ever had, and to tell you the truth, it was a gold star I wish I could have worn on my forehead.

But the best news was, it was over.

I was not prepared for the reception I got when I rounded to corner to where the bell was mounted. A dozen friends from the waiting room were poised to applaud and take pictures as I rang my way out of there. Pictures were taken with Kat and I, Chuck and Wie. I was truly touched at how much love and support you receive from not only staff but fellow patients and their families. Hooray for humanity. It again renewed my faith in the basic goodness of Americans and human kind in general.

We had thought about spending a quiet night in the apartment as our rent was paid up until Sunday, but the urge to be home was too great. We hit the apartment and our friends from Bakersfield showed up to help us pack. In no time the car was loaded and we bid goodbye to Houston. I was tired and didn't help much driving that first leg to Wichita Falls, but we made it, got a good room, and were on our way HOME.

Kat and I have always tried to come home a different way than we left, so this time we headed out to the Northeast corner of New Mexico, where there's some great hunting country I wanted to see, if only from the car, then north to Denver where we'd repeat our trip down until we reached Cheyenne, then our plan was to swing west and go home thorough Teton and Yellowstone National Parks. A bit of a treat on a trip we had to make anyway.

The second night we spent in Pueblo, Colorado, and took our time leaving the next morning as the traffic is so bad between Colorado Springs and Denver. We managed to miss most of it. We'd hoped to make it all the way to Dubois, Wyoming the third night, which would have meant only a little over three hundred miles for the last leg, but fate and some other folks bad karma intervened.

Twenty miles out of Cheyenne on Hwy. 80 we spotted smoke up ahead, and it was not long before we came to a standstill. Apparently three truck drivers a half mile ahead of us had also been paying too much attention to the smoke (which turned out to be a wrecked fuel truck on the other side of the highway) and one plowed into the rear of another, inviting a third to plow into his rear. It took three hours to extricate two drivers and a sleeper passenger from the wrecks. Both sides of the freeway were closed for hours.

At the risk of preaching, if I can tell you one more way to extend your life other than eating your fruits and vegetables, it's to not tailgate.

You'd think professional drivers would know better.

"I have found that if you love life, life will love you back."
--Arthur Rubinstein

31

WELL, I'M HOME. CAN'T BEGIN TO TELL YOU how good it feels to be in my own bed, my own shower, messing about in my own kitchen. Trying to get back in a normal routine of getting up, making herbal tea which used to be coffee, and hitting the machine to write for a while.

I'm a week post-last-treatment, and the bad news is the throat doesn't immediately start getting better. The radiation is a cumulative thing, and, in fact, the throat gets even more tender and it's become impossible to swallow. I'm down to 157 pounds which is college weight, and look a little like death warmed over...but hope we've actually beat that lurking monster into total submission.

Kat returned from town after visiting the muscle

store. I'm not sure if she actually went there to find some weight gain stuff for me or to look at all the buff boys who frequent the place, but I'll give her the benefit of the doubt. She came back with a gallon jug of Real Mass ®, "the complete weight gainer," rich vanilla milkshake. It's a dietary supplement. I made one, three scoops of powder to about sixteen ounces of milk or water. I used milk as if you've got to drink, it might as well be something that contributes to weight gain.

The boys and I are sighting in our rifles today, so I took the concoction along with me to the shooting range. I managed to get it down, as well as a half a banana and three Boosts ® so I managed to get over a thousand calories and over eighty grams of protein ingested. If I can keep that up I'll, hopefully, be able to maintain my weight. The next level of improvement is to gain weight. Of course, I could taste none of it, which makes it harder as eating's a chore rather than a pleasure.

One of the problems I've failed to mention, as it, like so many health issues is not one for polite conversation, is the bowel issue. You have a meeting at M. D. Anderson with a bowel specialist. Constipation or diarrhea is a constant problem when undergoing radiation. In my case it was constipation.

When you're consuming milk products and not much else, constipation is a problem. First off, your consumption of bulk is way down, and fiber almost non-existent. I finally quit visiting the bathroom except to produce a little urine, then after four days, and finally feeling as if I was sitting on a football, visited the pharmacy for a Fleet ® enema. It worked. I used three of them the last couple of weeks in Houston.

We attacked the problem with MiraLAX ®, a stool softener. It's mixed with water, which I'm supposed to drink anyway. The problem then became to balance the intake of MiraLax ® with the intake of Boost ®, Ensure ®, or Real Mass ®, so constipation didn't become diarrhea.

I'm glad this conversation is over.

This points to just one of the many patient services offered by M. D. Anderson. One of the most convenient to me, who is on the computer many hours a day, is myMDAnderson.com. You are given a number when you arrive and check in as a patient, and, among other things, it serves as your sign in to the webpage. Your appointments are all listed on the webpage and you have access to other services. You have the opportunity to attend pain seminars, bowel seminars, nutrition seminars, mental health seminars, and to visit specialists in any of those areas. There's transportation available, via busses, from all over the city. There's both valet and self-parking. There's childcare. They will provide you with names and contact information for other patients with the same diagnosis so if you just want to talk to someone in your same boat, you are able to do so. You're encouraged to bring your spouse or a friend along to treatments, so you'll have a hand to hold.

In addition to all this, there's a patient advocacy department, in case things are not going so well for you and you need someone to speak in your stead.

It's a most human place.

"Cancer is so limited. It cannot cripple love. It cannot corrode faith. It cannot eat away peace. It cannot shatter hope. It cannot destroy confidence. It cannot kill friendship. It cannot shutout memories. It cannot silence courage. It cannot invade the soul. It cannot reduce eternal life. It cannot quench the spirit."
--Author unknown

32

So, what is this monster, cancer?

Medusa should envy the many heads of this mutant miscreation.

There are over one hundred different types of cancer, classified by the type of cell it affects. The disease is the "out of control" growth of those cells when that cell's DNA goes awry. That "out of control" growth is what harms the body. Those cells form lumps, or tumors, except in the case of leukemia where cancer prevents normal cell functions.

Cells have a life cycle of their own, growth, division, and death. It's the abnormal growth of cells that is cancer—it's the abnormal life of the cell, that causes the death of the host. Normal cell death is called apoptosis, cancer cells have avoided this preprogrammed end. Tumors can impair every function of every system in the body. They can create chemical reactions that impair and interfere with the normal function of body systems.

Cancer moves through the blood stream or the lymph system, which is called metastasis. In my latest case, the primary tumor was believed to be at the base of the tongue, and metastasized to a lymph node in my neck, which was probably fortunate as the lump in the neck was how I discovered the problem.

Worldwide, in 2007, cancer claimed the lives of 7.6 million. And those are the ones we know of.

Cancer has touched, or will touch, us all. Early detection is a secret to survival. Gentlemen, take advantage of that free PSA blood test; ladies and gentlemen, of any cancer screening opportunity that comes along. Be proactive when you find a lump or find you have to urinate too often or are having trouble swallowing—or any abnormal bodily function or lack of function. Watch for those dark spots in your stool that may be blood, an indicator of colon cancer.

That annual physical becomes all-important, and make sure that includes a blood panel so your doc can identify any malfunction of your liver and other systems. I've had physical examinations from docs who would obviously have rather been somewhere else, and I've had good, complete, exams that made me feel the doc was truly into the oath he or she had taken. If you're not comfortable with your doc, find another.

Above all, if you are diagnosed with cancer, don't believe it's a death sentence. First off, you're doing the right thing or you wouldn't have discovered you had cancer in the first instance. You're being proactive by seeing the doc, by getting the biop he/she recommended. Knowing your enemy is halfway to destroying him, or it, in this case. Every year the rooster of cancer survivors grows and grows. One doc will look you in the eye and say you've got a 25% chance of making it five years (as has happened to me with both diagnosis) and another will say "we're going to whip this thing." Obviously, prefer to believe the one with the positive attitude, for you must maintain a positive attitude in order to allow your body to best fight this intruder.

Then attack, attack, attack. Live as healthy as you can, give your body all it needs to fight.

Kick ass.

You cannot be truthful if you are not courageous.
You cannot be loving if you are not courageous.
You cannot be trusting if you are not courageous.
You cannot enter into reality if you are not
courageous.
Hence courage comes first...
and everything else follows.

--Osho, Indian Spiritual Teacher

I READ SOMEWHERE THAT AN ACIDIC BODY IS A playground for cancer. Vegetables create an alkaline condition in the body. I've also read that your hypothalamus gland secretes acid when your angry or are thinking negatively, and alkaline when your happy and laughing. The gland is part of your brain, and its function is highly complex and complicated, and I'm not suggesting I begin to understand it. However, if the above is true, it's obvious that another of those old clichés, other than eat your vegetables, is true, and that's that laughter is the best medicine.

Mental health is such a large part of curing cancer. I truly believe that you are your own best doctor, or your own worst enemy. When you become dour and sour and believe that you're doomed, the odds are you are doomed. When anxiety drags you down its time to get up and come to your own emotional rescue. You must recognize that you've given up, or are giving up, and you, and only you, must take positive steps to change your train of thought. You must get that train on the right track. To do that you must accept that anxiety is a natural and normal part of the human psyche. Okay, I'm anxious. Okay, let's do something about it.

First and foremost you must accept that these are normal feelings. You've been dealt a tough hand. And as I've always said, when life gives you lemons, make lemonade. Accept your fate, and then work to do something about it. Give yourself permission to feel down and out, then give yourself permission to throw those feelings away. Cast them out and make room for positive thinking.

Deep breathing has always seemed to re-instill a feeling of life at its best for me, it's the very essence of life. When you begin feeling down, take a few deep breaths and tell yourself how good it feels to be alive, and that you're a long, long way from giving up.

Exercise is another elixir of life. Being able to move around and use your God-given body. Work up a sweat, tell yourself you're pushing the poisons out of your body, then enjoy the shower afterward.

Don't tune into Out of Africa when you need some laughs. Watch what you read, listen to, or watch in the way of entertainment. If the current political situation is stressful for you, to hell with it, find some old Abbott and Castello reruns. The country's going to go on for better or worse with or without your moaning over it.

Get a grip and focus on what you can do rather than what you can do nothing about. If cooking or canning or gardening makes you happy, then get out there and get your hands in the dirt.

Practice saying things in the positive. Drop the 't out of can't. It's I can, I will, I am, rather than the negative.

You're last thoughts of the night, after you've snuggled into the pillow should be, "I'm whipping this monster, I'm getting more and more healthy everyday. I'm going to live a long time and enjoy what's important to me: my wife, my husband, my children and my grandchildren, my friends. And this good night's sleep going to help with the battle."

Stay well, eat right, exercise, and live long.

The real test of courage is not to die...it's to live and fight on.

AFTERWORD

January 15, 2011

How many times did I wonder if I'd live to see another Christmas and New Year, to watch my grandchildren opening presents? How many times did I wonder if my grandson would get his first elk, or my son his first six point?

Well, here I am, and I've enjoyed those things mentioned above, and soooo much more since I was treated for cancer at M. D. Anderson.

Thank you, M. D. Anderson and the hospital your cotton trading money founded. What a gift to mankind? And thank you to the medical community of my home town, who I never doubted and who sent me off to Houston with the best possible backup.

Six months after being treated I went back to my excellent docs in Missoula, Montana, and was examined and poked and prodded and PET scanned, and was pronounced cancer free.

One can't help but celebrate, and one cannot help but take pause, as no one really knows what's going on in your body. It's said we continually have cancer cells traipsing around trying to make mischief, or worse. All we can do is do what we hope will give our body every opportunity to do its best.

In fighting the throat cancer, I set aside most of what I was doing to keep my PSA down, and now it's on the rise again, up to 01.49 as of yesterday. Nothing to get too excited about, but like all things heath it's something to be aware of and to kick in the teeth before it gets you down and stomps you.

So I'm back on the Chinese herbs, they've worked before and I'm confident they'll work again.

Since I wrote the main body of this journal I've lost two good friends to cancer...one actually passed from the results of a heart procedure, but he wsa being treated with chemo for prostate cancer, and probably was severely debilitated and may have lived a long life had he not been so. The other fought harder than anyone I've known to stay alive, and tried every alternative treatment known to him. Both were brave guys and both have a spot in my heart and always will. Go with God, Doug and John.

The rest of you, fight on, stay positive, and do what you can to help your body help the docs keep you healthy.

God bless you and all who fight to survive cancer, and all who fight to cure cancer.

March 15, 2013

CT scan of this date, still cancer FREE! ;-)

October 4, 2018

Still rocking and rolling. Hunting with my kids. Writing at least two books a year and several short stories. Working hard to see the country stays as I want it for children and grandchildren. God bless you and yours...stay assertive about your health. Visit me at ljmartin.com.

ABOUT THE AUTHOR

L. J. Martin is the author of over three dozen works of both fiction and non-fiction from Bantam, Avon, Pinnacle and his own Wolfpack Publishing. He lives in, and loves, Montana with his wife, NYT best-selling romantic suspense author Kat Martin. He's been a horse wrangler, cook as both avocation and vocation, volunteer firefighter, real estate broker, general contractor, appraiser, disaster evaluator for FEMA, and traveled a good part of the world, some in his own ketch. A hunter, fisherman, photographer, cook, father and grandfather, he's been car and plane wrecked, visited a number of jusgados and a road camp, and survived cancer twice. He carries a bail-enforcement, bounty hunter, shield. He knows about what he writes about, and tries to write about what he knows.

Made in the USA
Middletown, DE
16 July 2019